The Real Benefits

of

Exercise

Other books available include:

Motivation, Achievement & Challenges

Understanding & Building Confidence

Managing Stress & Preventing Depression

How to Sleep Better!

Weight Loss & Healthy Eating

Please make a donation if you can

TEXT: BOOK32£5

To: 70070

Or an online donation via:

www.justgiving.com/healthbooks

www.cymhealth.org

THANK YOU!

The Real Benefits

of

Exercise

by

Charlie Wardle

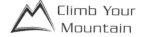
Climb Your Mountain

Published under licence by Brown Dog Books and

The Self Publishing Partnership

7 Green Park Station, Bath BA1 1JB

www.selfpublishingpartnership.co.uk

ISBN book: 978-1-903056-95-0

ISBN e-book: 978-1-903056-96-7

Cover design by Kevin Rylands

Printed and bound by CPI Group (UK) Ltd, Croydon CR0 4YY

Contents

Part 3 – Exercise and Activity Options 57

Part 4 – How to Get Motivated to Exercise 65

About the author

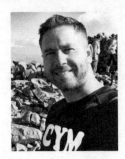

Charlie Wardle founded the Climb Your Mountain (CYM) charity in 2008 with the objective of helping as many people as possible to climb the personal mountain they may face in their life for whatever reason. CYM provides a wide range of both educational and physical activity opportunities so that people can help themselves to a healthier and happier life. Previously, Charlie had a successful finance, accounting and marketing career with a number of large blue-chip companies. He is a qualified Chartered Accountant (ACA) and has an MBA from Cranfield School of Management. His passion is health, wellbeing and fitness.

The education and learning side, called CYM Health, offers a range of free health and wellbeing books, courses, workshops, videos, talks and advice which are written, delivered and presented by Charlie. He has spent the last few years researching, reading, thinking, discussing and meeting with hundreds of people in order to build up the knowledge and experience that is then offered to others.

Please read the section at the end of this book to find out more about the Climb Your Mountain (CYM) charity and also please visit the website www.climbyourmountain.org for an online video workshop focusing on this book. Plus make sure you read the other health and wellbeing books in this series.

Introduction

'Warning: Exercise can seriously improve your health and happiness!'

Pretty much everyone is aware that exercise is good for us and most people will be able to give you some good reasons why exercise and physical activity is beneficial. However, there are probably far more benefits to exercise than most people realise, and through knowing and understanding more of the real benefits hopefully people will be encouraged and motivated to be more physically active and therefore to improve their health and happiness.

This book is designed to provide a wide range of information that details the real benefits of exercise in all its different ways. I have tried to write the book in an easy-to-read and practical format and it is aimed at anyone and everyone, no matter their age, sex, background or current activity levels.

Our health is and should be extremely important to us all, yet as society develops, technology advances and we have more choices, one of the issues is that people, on the whole, are doing less exercise and are less physically active than previous generations. This is contributing towards growing health issues that could be prevented. Exercise provides so many benefits to our physical, mental and emotional health in a variety of ways and should not be seen as a luxury or a low priority in our lives. If we can make it a higher priority and incorporate it into our lives on a regular basis then we can all benefit and improve our health and happiness.

As the book will show, exercise and physical activity are natural for humans and we have developed and evolved very successfully as a species due to our athletic and physical abilities. Exercise is also very accessible, as there is such a wide range of options and opportunities no matter who you are. It is probably the most effective, accessible and natural way to help with issues such as stress, depression, anxiety, lack of confidence and low self-esteem. It is one of the best ways to prevent, manage and overcome physical health issues too, and although at times doing exercise may seem like the harder choice to make, it will reward you with so many benefits that the effort is always worth it.

So, no matter what your current situation is, you can benefit from being more physically active and doing exercise, building up how much you do, improving your fitness, stamina, strength and conditioning. You can feel better about yourself, increase your confidence, meet new people, try new things, go to new places, lose weight, tone up, prevent illness and improve your overall health and, of course, feel happier as a result!

What is exercise and how do we define it?

Formal definitions:

Exercise – activity requiring physical effort, carried out to sustain or improve health and fitness.

Exercise – a planned, structured, and repetitive activity for the purpose of improving or maintain physical fitness.

Exercise is a form of physical activity and 'physical activity' can be defined as any movement of the body that requires energy expenditure (this energy expenditure is usually measured in kilocalories). This includes any movement through the day, excluding sitting still or lying down. For example, walking to class, taking the stairs, mowing the lawn, and even cleaning your house can be considered physical activity. Exercise is a type of physical activity, but not every physical activity is exercise.

In this book we focus on exercise, but also include other areas of physical activity, as pretty much any type of physical activity will have benefits to us and should therefore also be encouraged and discussed. Unfortunately there is a growing trend of people doing less and less exercise and being less and less physically active, not just in the UK but across the world.

Physical inactivity is now identified as the fourth leading risk factor for global mortality, causing an estimated 3.2 million deaths globally (approx 6%) according to the World Health Organisation (WHO). This follows high blood pressure (13%), tobacco use (9%) and high blood glucose (6%). Overweight and obesity are responsible for 5% of global mortality. Physical inactivity levels are rising in many countries, with major implications for the prevalence of noncommunicable diseases (NCDs) and the general health of the population worldwide.

In the UK, the situation is pretty bleak, with 12.5 million people in England alone failing to achieve 30 minutes of moderate-intensity physical activity per week; physical inactivity currently accounts for nearly one-fifth of premature deaths in the UK. With projections showing that inactivity levels are due to increase by a further 15 per cent by 2030 there is no doubt that the issue requires immediate national attention and urgent action.

Lord Sebastian Coe, who was head of the London Olympics and Paralympics, has said:

> *'Turning the tide of inactivity would be a hugely important outcome for our legacy story, which would have a massive long-term impact on our nation's health and wellbeing. Supporting people that do little or no daily activity to become a bit more active is where the biggest public health gains can be made and the maximum financial returns on public investment attained. Turning the tide of physical inactivity must be viewed as a national priority.'*

A few facts

From Public Health England from their Everybody Active, Every Day campaign (2014)

- More than 1 in 17 adults in the UK are living with diabetes. Being active can reduce the risk of developing this illness by 30-40%.

- If being active was a pill we would be rushing to prescribe it. Physical activity is essential for health and reduces the risk of many preventable diseases and conditions from cancer to depression.

- Physical inactivity is responsible for 1 in 6 deaths in the UK, making it as dangerous as smoking. But over 1 in 4 of us take less than 30 minutes of physical activity each week.

- Inactive people have three times the rate of moderate to severe depression compared to active people. Being active is central to our mental health and feelings of general wellbeing.

- The estimated cost to the UK every year of physical inactivity is £7.4bn.

Questionnaires

Before writing the book I sent out a questionnaire to a mix of people (young and old, male and female, fit and unfit, etc.) and asked them the following four questions related to exercise and physical activity. Over the next few pages there is a selection of real answers from real people, which I felt were representative of the general population.

What prevents you from doing exercise?
What are the factors as to why don't you exercise?

- *Depression and a lack of motivation associated with that.*

- *Fitting it in to my daily routine can sometimes make exercise difficult. I am at my best around midday so try and do my exercise then. If the weather is horrible I won't exercise outside.*

- *My brain struggles to switch off to exercise... I keep thinking of the work I should be doing.*

- *Childcare limitations; injury; having the time.*

- *Lack of motivation and lack of energy.*

- *Not having anyone to go with, would rather not go alone.*

- *If the weather is particularly bad I won't take the dogs out for a walk.*

- *Time, feeling tired, people to train with, lack of motivation.*

What do you dislike about doing exercise/activities?

- *Nothing nowadays. I used to feel very self-conscious, which was a reason not to go to a gym.*

- *Being depressed was a factor in not having the motivation or energy to exercise; however, finding something I enjoy and initially having someone to go with to encourage me was really important and helpful.*

- *I don't like doing too much of the same thing as I get bored. This is the reason I do running, walking and karate. It gives me some variety. I change running routes and training plans, for example may do hill training one day, 5k another day, fartlek another day.*

- *I struggle with time out specifically for the gym as my brain won't switch off to what needs to be completed at work; I suppose that boils down to, rightly or wrongly, me feeling my time could be spent better doing other things.*

- *Monetary cost.*

- *If it's cold or wet outside it's not as enjoyable!*

- *The hassle of changing, going to gym, showering, etc. Sometimes the cost.*

When you do exercise what are your main reasons for doing it? Why do you exercise?

- *Every day I do something. Hotpod Yoga at least 3 times a week and Bootcamp type exercises at home based on a Bootcamp I used to attend (that no longer runs).*

- *Walks with other people and weekends with groups away are great.*

- *I do it all as it makes me feel fitter, stronger and more confident than ever before.*

- *I exercise mostly in lunch breaks, but do also exercise three evenings a week. Exercise makes me feel good. It makes me feel healthy and happy. Depending on the type of exercise, it can help me forget about all the stresses I may be having at the time. On the other hand if I'm out running, it allows me time to reflect on what I am doing at the time. I often find answers to work-related problems whilst out running.*

- *I actually enjoy the classes – Body Pump, Step, Zumba, etc.*

- *If I feel I need to tone up and it makes me feel good.*

- *When I've set a goal such as a 10k race and then need to train.*

- *To keep active, to maintain healthy weight, to get fresh air. As I get older I am very much aware of how important it is to keep supple and flexible, and practise yoga regularly with a personal yoga teacher who makes the work fun and jolly hard!*

- *Walking is my main method of exercise and I do this to take the dogs out.*

- *To keep in shape, to feel healthy, to look good, enjoy the challenge, knowing it's good for you, meeting different people.*

What do you enjoy about doing exercise/activities?

- *The large number of new friends I have made in the last year since being more active. I feel fitter, stronger and more confident than ever before. Having gained this through the physical activity and this new support network has enabled me to resolve my self-esteem issues to such an extent that the life challenges I now face e.g. a recent romantic 'failure', means I am able to deal with this is in a very pragmatic and much stronger manner.*

- *I love the way it makes me feel. Like I said before, depending on the type of exercise it can give me time out to reflect on things but on the other hand it can also help block things out and gives me something to focus on.*

- *I like the social side that comes with it too; with all my exercise I am part of a group. This helps encourage you to continue the exercise but you also get to meet people with similar interests as you.*

- *That once the class starts I know I will see it through – I wouldn't walk out early.*

- *I know I am terribly unfit – I don't like that feeling, if I attend a class the challenge getting through it and the feeling of improving class on class is a great sense of achievement... i.e. after a few classes I can raise the step to the higher level or cope with greater weights etc.*

- *The 'Me' time it gives me.*

- *I can think more clearly, it clears my head. It makes me feel happy.*

- *Psychologically, it makes me feel better physically and mentally. Not being one to sit in front of a screen, I much prefer, and enjoy, being outdoors.*

- *Seeing the wildlife; birds, plants/flowers opening up etc. etc.*

- *The feel-good factor, looking good, challenging myself and achieving goals.*

Human evolution – born to be active

'Your body can stand almost anything; it's your mind that you have to convince.'

There is so much evidence in many different forms to indicate that we are healthier and happier if we exercise; exercise can come in so many ways and just about everyone can find some activity they can do and hopefully enjoy. However, often people associate exercise with running, and most people in modern times unfortunately don't run and are horrified at the thought! They are too unfit, overweight, not used to running, don't find it appealing, can't get motivated, can't run very far or very fast and it is simply easier not to bother. And why should we bother when we have cars, trains, buses, bikes, etc. for transport? We no longer have to go hunting for food so we just drive or occasionally walk to the shops. We are very rarely put in positions of danger where we have to run from something or towards something for our safety. There just isn't the need to run, so why bother?

Well, another way to look at this apart from everything that will be said on the benefits is to show how humans are natural athletes and we are literally born to run. Unlike any other animal on the planet we have evolved into the most intelligent, superior species. That has happened for a number of reasons including the very important ability to run like no other creature.

There are so many features and unique qualities to the human body that seem to show clearly that we were born to run. For example, we have an Achilles tendon that is only needed for running. Why do we have this unless we were designed to run, and why do we have arches on our feet with small toes to allow us to run whereas chimps and monkeys don't have Achilles tendons or arches, just flat feet with very long toes designed for walking and climbing? We have a nuchal ligament in the back of our neck to support our head and balance it, which is only needed for running. Dogs, cats and horses have a nuchal ligament to help them run but again chimps and monkeys do not. Humans also have big bottoms, which are very helpful for running yet have no benefit for walking. Next time you see a chimp look at how small their bottoms are compared to humans.

A further unique feature of humans is our lack of a tail. No other running animal or two-legged creature has no tail. The way we balance while at speed is the added combination of the nuchal ligament in the neck and the fact that our head is heavy compared to other animals. This heavy weight on the top of our upright position provides support and balance, allowing us to move at speed for long distances without wasting too much energy.

We are upright creatures with features that are otherwise only found on our four-legged animal friends renowned for their running and speed. Yet, unlike horses, dogs, cats, deer, etc., the rhythm of our breathing is not directly related to our movement. Watch a leopard run across the African plains and its breathing is directly related to its strides; as its legs stretch out its lungs open and when the legs close together with the stride the lungs contract like bellows. So while the leopard's breathing is matched with its running stride, humans' breathing is different, as we will typically do at least two strides to one breath.

Another very important feature and strong advantage is the number of sweat glands we have. No other creature has as many and can sweat so much. This ability to sweat helps us to keep cool for much longer. So although many animals can run faster than us, they cannot sustain it for very long before they overheat and have to stop or slow down significantly. If you take a dog out on a hot day and they run and run, they will eventually just stop, much earlier than a fit and healthy human would do.

There is an annual horse versus man race over a 50-mile distance. Most people would never dream that a human could beat a horse in a running race, yet most years the humans come out victorious. Animals just don't have the endurance that humans have because they cannot sweat and keep cool for long periods. Humans have the best air-cooled engine of any animal and are able to run for hours at a time if necessary. Something else that might surprise you is that humans have a longer running stride than a horse. If you record and slow down the footage of a running horse then you will see that each leg has a relatively small stride, and the energy required to run fast with all four legs like that is significantly more than for a human. So whereas a horse can go at a much faster rate for about 10 minutes, it soon slows down to a slower pace than a strong long-distance human runner.

Unlike most sports and activities running is age-friendly. What I mean by that is that humans can go on running until they would be considered very old, without losing much of their ability compared to their younger years. A large study was made of marathon runners and it was shown that if you take the average best times for someone at 19 years of age and compare those across the age range then humans reach their peak in terms of running ability after 8 years, at the age of 27. The subsequent decline in ability is significantly slower than the time it took to reach the peak. Not until age 64 does a human's ability fall back to their ability at age 19. So 8 years of improving and 37 years of gradual decline. In many ways this shows that 'you don't stop running because you get old – you get old because you stop running'!

Something else to consider and observe at the opposite end of the scale is how young children are so naturally active. They can seemingly go for hours playing, running, jumping and being active and it looks so normal and natural. The reason is that it is natural and normal for children to be active and enjoy being active, and this should be encouraged for as long as possible. Before computer games and televisions, children would spend much of their time actively playing, using up energy, running about and enjoying the natural freedom and benefits it brings.

As children get older they generally become less physically active and that seems to be for three main reasons. Firstly, there are so many alternatives these days, especially what we can do with computers, games and televisions, and it is easier to encourage children to use these as it requires less effort and is easier for parents to manage. Secondly, as a consequence of many factors, including poor diet and nutrition, worsening sleep habits, more stress, and health and safety issues, children lack motivation, are more tired and have fewer opportunities to play, exercise, play sport and be physically active. Finally, we do not appreciate the benefits of exercise, nor are we fully aware of the health risks and consequences of not exercising, because of a lack of education, training and learning.

If children were encouraged to keep being active, as they do so well naturally when they are younger, then more of them would benefit and be healthier and happier. If there was more education, with more opportunities and more emphasis placed on exercise and activity it would benefit us all.

Part 1

Why Do We Not Exercise?

There are many reasons and factors as to why we don't exercise or why the levels of physical activity have fallen so much in recent decades. Below are some of the factors that may apply:

We don't need to any more – choices

Most of us who live in a modern developed country like the UK do not have to exercise or be active if we choose not to. We can choose to stay at home the whole time and order in food or have groceries and other shopping delivered to us. If we do leave the house we can use our car to drive to wherever we are going, be that work, shopping, to see family and friends, etc. Exercise or physical activity is not compulsory in modern life. It has become an option that we can choose if we wish, but it is no longer something we have to do or need to do and therefore it is a choice.

Many people, if they have a choice between driving to work or walking to work, will choose the car option. If they had a choice between going to the gym for a workout or sitting at home watching a film they would choose the film option. If they had the choice between using an elevator or walking up three flights of stairs they would use the lift option.

In the past, these options would not exist or wouldn't be so prevalent, so people would naturally do more exercise and be more physically active. Additionally, as the younger generations do less and less exercise and spend more hours playing computer games than physical games, it becomes more the norm and accepted that exercise is a choice rather than a necessity.

Too busy – not enough time

Our modern lives are often very busy and hectic with lots of pressures, expectations and responsibilities. It can often feel we are chasing our own tail at times and we just don't have enough time to do everything we need to do, let alone additional activities like exercising. Because most people now see exercise as an option and an additional extra that isn't a necessity, we tend to put it lower down on our priority list.

Going to work, cleaning the house, doing the shopping, taking the kids to school, seeing family and friends, etc., all too often become a much higher priority than exercising, and most of us feel tired much of the time, so then to try and exercise as well becomes even more difficult.

> *'I don't <u>find</u> the time to exercise... I <u>make</u> the time to exercise.'*

Too tired

It seems that most of us often feel tired for much of the time, and exercise has even less appeal when we don't have the energy. Feeling tired can be the result of many factors, which generally tend to be more modern-day lifestyle reasons such as increased stress, higher depression rates, being overweight, obesity issues, lack of sleep or poor-quality sleep, poor nutrition, alcohol consumption, drug-related issues and other factors that can make us lethargic.

Even though exercise is very likely to provide you with more energy, help you sleep better, reduce stress and depression, help you lose weight, encourage you to drink less and eat more healthily, etc., it becomes very difficult to choose to do exercise when you are feeling tired.

Sleep is a big issue for many people, and the average amount of sleep people now get is only 6 hours and 35 minutes each night. Without sufficient sleep people will be more tired and lethargic, lacking the energy and motivation to do exercise, and will more often resort to the easier choice of not exercising. In addition, what people eat and drink plays a major role in how they feel and their energy levels, or lack of energy.

You may find two further books in this series, *How to Sleep Better!* and *Weight Loss & Healthy Eating* (available from Amazon and iBooks and iTunes), helpful on these topics.

Too expensive

Although there are numerous different ways to exercise and do physical activities at no cost or very minimal cost, there is often a perception that to do more exercise will cost money and be too expensive. Especially given the fact that many people and families do not have much disposable income, when exercise is viewed as an extra or even a luxury it is often pushed back down the list of things to do because it is not a necessity, whereas other things are or are perceived to be.

Of course, some activities, sports and forms of exercise can be expensive and that then becomes a barrier, but there are so many forms of exercise that are not costly and the benefits you get in return hugely outweigh any associated costs. The question should be asked 'What value do you put on your health?' How much would you spend on products like creams, moisturisers, make-up, hair products, beauty treatments, supplements, clothes, shoes, etc.? Compare this to how much you would spend or invest on your health through exercise and physical activity.

Not fit enough

Many people shy away from exercise, activities or sports because they feel they would not be able to take part given their current fitness level or health. This may be true of certain activities or sports, but there are many forms of exercise that can be done by anyone at any fitness level and then it is all about progressing. The human body is remarkable in so many ways, including how quickly it will adapt and progress, and your fitness level and capabilities will improve exponentially if you are sensible and stick with it.

It shouldn't matter what your starting position is, focus on improving and progressing steadily and you will. Also, many people underestimate their fitness levels; just because they haven't walked for three hours before doesn't mean they couldn't do it if they had to or chose to try.

> *'If you want something you never had... You have to do something you've never done.'*

Don't enjoy it

Many people will say they do not enjoy exercise or sport and will believe that this is so, which means they are unlikely to do much or try anything. It may well be the case that many people do not enjoy certain activities, but there are so many possibilities and things to try that I am sure there are physical activities that everyone can enjoy to some degree.

Also, although it helps to enjoy something, it doesn't have to be enjoyable for you to do it. We do many things on a daily, weekly, monthly or yearly basis that we don't enjoy but we have to do or we know is beneficial for us. For example, many people don't enjoy going to the dentist but they still go!

No one to exercise with

For some people a reason for not exercising can be that they have no one else to exercise with or to join them in a particular activity. This could be a factor in some sports or activities where you need someone else or it could be a safety issue. However, you have to take some personal responsibility. Many forms of exercise can be done alone, or you can often find other people to exercise with by making a bit of effort or research, or by asking friends, family and colleagues if they will participate with you.

There are many running clubs, walking groups, cycling clubs, dance classes, fitness groups, gyms, etc., which can be free or very low cost, where there will be other people for you to exercise with who are often in a similar position to yourself. So do some research, make some enquiries and go for it. You are also likely to make some new friends, too, as a result.

Don't know what to do or where to go

Many people are not sure what sort of exercise or activity they should be doing or how to do it. There are so many options, but many will be untried by them and they may then be hesitant, apprehensive or not sure how to start. They may fancy trying something but don't know where to go or what it may entail.

To a degree this is understandable and if doing exercise or sport is not familiar to you then it can be a bit daunting. However, there is plenty of information available online or from clubs, groups, gyms, sports centres etc., and many people who are willing to offer advice and provide further information and help. You are likely to be pleasantly surprised if you research the information or ask for help regarding what to do and where to go.

No motivation

Lacking motivation is often a big factor in why people don't exercise or don't do as much as they want to or should do. We have looked at various factors above that could lower motivation or have a negative impact on your desire to exercise, and there are usually many reasons or issues that contribute to poor motivation.

There is a section later in the book called 'How to get motivated to exercise', which hopefully will help and make a difference, so you become more motivated and then participate in more exercise and physical activity, which in turn should increase motivation further.

Stress, depression and anxiety

Rates of conditions like stress, depression and anxiety continue to increase and they can also have a big impact on the levels of exercise and activity people do. Although exercise is very beneficial for these conditions, people who are experiencing them will often do less activity, as some of the symptoms can include lack of motivation, tiredness, poor diet, lack of sleep, low confidence, being more withdrawn and lack of desire.

Given some of those symptoms it is not surprising that people with such conditions tend to do less exercise and physical activity, and if the rates are increasing then even fewer people will be active. One of the best ways to manage, treat and prevent stress, depression and anxiety is to exercise; this is explored in the following chapters.

You might find another book in this series, *Managing Stress & Preventing Depression,* of benefit here.

Food and diet

Our modern diet is generally very poor and continues to worsen, especially with the increasing volume of processed foods and sugar-rich products. Also, in developed countries, on average we consume far more food and therefore calories than we need and that we use for energy. And as more and more people become overweight this often leads to them doing less and less exercise.

If you are overweight and eating an unhealthy diet you are less likely to exercise for several reasons. You are more likely to feel tired and lack the energy and motivation to put the additional effort into physical activities and exercise. Many people feel unfit and do not think they can do the exercises others may be doing, so tend to shy away. Also, many overweight people are self-conscious and don't want to feel out of place if the exercise is with others or where other people can see them.

It is not just people who are overweight that are affected by their food and diet when it comes to exercise. Many people who are not overweight still eat unhealthily and do not consume the good foods that provide energy and motivation. Too much sugar and salt, and too many carbohydrates, starches and processed foods tend to make you feel lethargic, and only provide energy boosts for a very short time before making you feel tired again.

If you ate a lot more vegetables, salad, fruit, complex carbohydrates and lean protein, and cut out the sugars, breads, fats and processed foods you would have much more energy, be more positive, more motivated and maintain a good, healthy weight.

For more information on this area, there is another book available in this series called *Weight Loss & Healthy Eating*.

Part 2

The Benefits of Exercise

Physiological and mental health benefits

'To keep the body in good health is a duty...otherwise we shall not be able to keep our mind strong and clear.' – Buddha

Effects on brain chemistry

We all know that exercise is good for us and can improve our health and make us feel better, yet most of us don't actually know why. The main reason is that exercise makes our brain function at its best. Physical activity is crucial to the way we think and feel, and plays a significant role in regulating and improving our neurotransmitters and bolstering our brain's infrastructure. The brain responds like most muscles do by growing with use and withering with inactivity. The neurons in the brain connect to each other like leaves on branches, and exercise causes those branches to grow and bloom with new buds, thus enhancing and improving our brain function.

The brain is, of course, very complex and much of what goes on is still not really understood. However, it is know that many of our thoughts, behaviours and emotions are controlled by chemicals in the brain called neurotransmitters and four key neurotransmitters are:

Serotonin – is responsible for mood, anxiousness, self-esteem and impulsive and compulsive behaviour.

Beta-endorphin – is responsible for modulating emotional and physical pain. It contributes to feelings of self-esteem, euphoria and emotional confidence.

Norepinephrine – affects arousal, alertness, attention and mood.

Dopamine – is vital to movement, attention, cognition, motivation and pleasure (and addiction).

Ideally, we would all have regulated and optimal levels of these neurotransmitters so we feel happy, well balanced and confident, and our thoughts, behaviours and emotions are how we would like them to be and regarded as 'normal'. However, for many people this is not the case and their neurotransmitters are lower than optimal and poorly regulated, leading to a range of emotional and mental health issues which also affect physical health.

Exercise and physical activity is a fantastic way of helping to elevate and regulate these chemicals and make us happier, more alert, less stressed, less anxious, more balanced, less reactive, etc. Our brain will respond very quickly to exercise and positive results and outcomes can be seen immediately, as well as continued and sustained benefits. Our brain is so important and should be given the respect and attention that is necessary, and the good news is that exercise can be incredibly effective for our brain and therefore for our overall health and wellbeing. Do not underestimate what exercise can do for your brain!

'Exercise is a wonder drug that hasn't been bottled.'

Improved learning, memory and cognitive behaviour

Exercise increases the level of brain chemicals called growth factors, which help make new brain cells and establish new connections between brain cells to help us learn and improve our memory. Interestingly, complicated activities like playing tennis or taking a dance class provide the biggest brain boost, as you are challenging your brain even more when you have to think about coordination. Like muscles, you have to stress your brain cells to get them to be more active and to grow.

Complicated activities also improve our capacity to learn by enhancing our attention and concentration skills, according to German researchers who found that high-school students scored better on high-attention tasks after doing 10 minutes of a complicated fitness routine compared to those doing 10 minutes of regular activity, and those who hadn't exercised at all scored the worst.

The benefits of exercise come directly from its ability to reduce insulin resistance, reduce inflammation, and stimulate the release of the growth factors mentioned, which are chemicals in the brain that affect the health of brain cells, the growth of new blood vessels in the brain, and even the abundance and survival of new brain cells. Researchers also found that regular aerobic exercise, the kind that gets your heart and your sweat glands pumping, appears to boost the size of the hippocampus, the brain area involved in verbal memory and learning.

Exercise helps memory and thinking through indirect means, too, as physical activity can improve mood and sleep, and reduce stress and anxiety; problems in these areas frequently cause or contribute to cognitive impairment. So if you want to improve your alertness, learning ability and memory and reduce your risk of cognitive decline and potentially associated conditions like dementia then be more active, because this exercises the brain as well as the body.

Stress

A recent survey published by the Mental Health Foundation in the UK found that 59% of British adults felt their life was more stressful than it was five years ago. 47% of all survey respondents said they felt stressed every day and a further 24% said they felt stressed every few days. The Health and Social Care Information Centre also recently published data which showed hospital admissions for stress have risen by 7% in just 12 months, and the Health and Safety Executive recently published figures which indicate a rise in sick days due to work-related stress.

Stress causes the body to produce more of the so-called 'fight or flight' chemicals which prepare it for an emergency. Adrenaline and noradrenaline raise blood pressure and increase heart rate and perspiration. They can also reduce blood flow to the skin and reduce stomach activity. The body produces cortisol which in turn causes fat and sugar to be released into the bloodstream (but also reduces the efficiency of the immune system). All these changes are the body's way of making it easier to fight or run away. Unfortunately these changes are less helpful for individuals stuck in a busy office or on an overcrowded train. They cannot fight and cannot run away. Because of this, they cannot use up the chemicals their own bodies have produced to protect them.

Over time these chemicals and the changes they produce can cause serious damage to health. For example, people suffering from stress may start to experience headaches, nausea and indigestion. They may breathe more quickly, perspire more, have palpitations or suffer from various aches and pains. Longer-term stress can lead to feelings of strain, worry, insomnia and exhaustion, and increased risk of health problems such as heart attacks and strokes. The Mental Health Foundation survey found that 18% of people found drinking alcohol helpful for stress and 10% found smoking helpful, while only 6% would consider visiting a GP. This is worrying because in the long run alcohol and smoking can make mental and physical health problems much worse.

Physical activity can be very helpful in reducing or managing stress. Cross-sectional studies on adults who are employed have found that highly active individuals tend to have lower stress rates compared to low active individuals. Several mechanisms have been suggested to explain how physical activity may reduce the harmful effects of stress. These include that physical activity reduces arousal (i.e. enhances mood due to distraction from worries or biochemical changes) or increases positive health behaviours during periods of stress (i.e. decreased smoking and healthier eating habits). It has also been suggested that the higher levels of fitness brought about by physical activity result in more efficient stress regulation (i.e. reduced secretion of hormones, lowered blood pressure) or enhanced recovery from stress.

Depression

Depression varies from mild to severe, and between 8% and 12% of the British population experience diagnosed depression in any one year. In recent years prescription rates for antidepressant medication have increased significantly. However, antidepressants are not equally effective for everyone, and many people are reluctant to take antidepressants for long periods, often because of their side effects, a situation that can lead to non-compliance with medication or not seeking treatment. Psychological therapies (e.g. cognitive behavioural therapy or CBT) have become more widely available but there are often long waiting lists for free or low-cost services.

Exercise can be an alternative treatment for depression as well as helping to manage and prevent the condition. It can be used as a stand-alone treatment approach or in combination with medication and/or psychological therapy. It has very few side effects, if any, and does not have the stigma that some people perceive to be attached to taking antidepressants or attending counselling. In addition physical activity is available to all, has few costs attached and is an empowering approach that can support self-management.

The majority of published trials have found a positive outcome for physical activity in treating depression where they have used aerobic physical activity and were supervised. Furthermore, all modes of physical activity and locations (e.g. home or gym) were equally effective, although it is noteworthy here that outdoor locations were not studied as these provide access to sunlight and green open spaces. Effective intervention programmes were supervised, but whether the supervisor was an exercise professional or from some other professional background did not have an impact on their effectiveness. Both group and individual physical activity programmes were found to be equally effective.

Implications of the above studies are that meeting the recommended public health guidelines for physical activity seems to offer greater benefits compared to lower levels of physical activity. Individuals' preferences about physical activity type (e.g. swimming, dancing and football) can and should be accommodated into physical activity programmes. Personal preferences of participants with regard to physical activity location and whether to be active in groups or individually should also be considered. Furthermore research suggests that exercising at preferred intensity results in greater reductions in depression compared to exercising at a prescribed intensity. In other words, when people are given choice and control over the physical activity, they do report greater benefits to their mental health.

Anxiety

As with depression, anxiety symptoms can vary from mild to severe. Feeling anxious is sometimes perfectly normal. However, people with generalised anxiety disorder find it hard to control their worries; their feelings of anxiety are more constant and often affect their daily life. Generalised anxiety disorder affects at least 5% of adults in the UK. Other conditions where anxiety is the main symptom include panic disorder, phobias and post-traumatic stress disorder. Anxiety often occurs alongside depression, i.e. people often experience both problems at the same time. Treatments for anxiety include anxiolytic medication and psychological therapy. Limitations to the use of medication and psychological therapy in the treatment of anxiety are similar to the limitations to their use to treat depression.

Also similar to the treatment of depression, there is mounting evidence that physical activity is beneficial as a treatment for people with both mild and severe (clinical) anxiety. A review of 19 studies, which had investigated the effect of physical activity on healthy adults, found that increasing physical activity in this group resulted in reduced anxiety. Further analyses of these studies revealed that interventions were most effective when: participants engaged in moderate or high-intensity physical activity; physical activity was supervised; the intervention was delivered to individuals (rather than group-based); and when participants were encouraged to continue exercising at a fitness centre following the intervention (rather than at home).

Less is known about the effect of exercise on specific severe types of anxiety, such as panic attacks, social anxiety disorder, generalised anxiety disorder or post-traumatic stress disorder. However, data do show there are lower rates of clinical anxiety amongst people who are active than people who are not and intervention studies have shown exercise holds promise for reducing symptoms of clinical anxiety. For example, one study compared patients with various types of clinical anxiety who were randomly assigned to CBT plus home-based walking, or CBT plus additional education sessions. Patients in the home-based walking group reported significantly greater reductions in anxiety, depression and stress following treatment compared to those receiving CBT without exercise. Several other small-scale studies have focused on a particular type of anxiety (e.g. panic disorder or post-traumatic stress disorder) and shown positive effects for exercise in reducing anxiety symptoms in these groups of patients.

Confidence and self-esteem

Self-esteem is a key indicator of psychological wellbeing. People with high self-esteem tend to have high life satisfaction, resilience and greater achievement in education and work. On the other hand low self-esteem tends to be associated with mental illness, anxiety and hopelessness. Self-esteem can be defined as the sum of a person's perceptions of their competence in several areas of their life; for example, academic, emotional, social and physical. Of these areas the physical aspect of self-esteem (i.e. one's competence regarding stamina, strength, sport ability and body attractiveness) has been shown to have a strong influence on overall self-esteem.

Physical activity is a behaviour which has a strong influence on physical self-esteem and a smaller but significant influence on overall self-esteem. Studies have found that people who participate in physical activity typically have greater physical and overall self-esteem. This relationship has been found in children, adolescents, young adults, adults and older people, and across both males and females.

A review of 113 physical activity studies found three factors that influenced how much impact physical activity interventions have on a person's self-esteem. The greatest gains in self-esteem occurred for people who initially had low self-esteem, those whose fitness increased during the intervention, and those who were active on more days per week. All types of physical activity were equally effective at increasing self-esteem. Overall the researchers concluded from their review that physical activity interventions which aim to increase self-esteem should include physical activity that is moderately demanding and lasts for 12 weeks or more.

As all types of physical activity have been found to be equally effective, people should choose a type of physical activity based on what they enjoy doing. Another important factor to consider when using physical activity to enhance self-esteem is that physical activity should provide opportunities to experience feelings of accomplishment. Physical activity goals should be set so that they are achievable and result in feelings of success. For this to be achieved the duration, type, intensity and frequency of physical activity in any programme should be set in relation to an individual's physical fitness and previous physical activity experience.

Dementia and cognitive decline in older people

Increasing life expectancy and a growing population of people aged over 65 has led to an increase in the number of people living with dementia and cognitive decline. Dementia affects some 800,000 people in the UK, and the number of people with the condition is steadily increasing because people are living longer. It is estimated that by 2020, the number of people with dementia in the UK will have increased to around one million. With no known cure, ways to improve the lives of those living with the condition are vital.

The main symptom of dementia is memory loss; it is a progressive disease which results in people becoming more impaired over time. Decline in cognitive functions such as attention and concentration also occurs in older people, including those who do not go on to develop dementia.

Physical activity can protect people against developing dementia and for people who have already developed the disease can delay further declines in functioning. Studies show that adults participating in daily physical activity have a 20-30% lower risk for dementia. Physical activity also seems to reduce the likelihood of experiencing cognitive decline in people who do not go on to develop dementia.

Exercise throughout a person's life plays a significant role in reducing the risk of developing dementia, a study spanning 35 years has found. The Cardiff University study, which began with 2,235 men from Caerphilly in 1979, found factors including diet and not smoking had an impact on preventing illnesses developing in older age. However, exercise had the single biggest influence on dementia levels. People in the study who fulfilled four of these factors had a 60% decrease in dementia and cognitive decline rates, with exercise named as the strongest mitigating factor. The study was funded by the Medical Research Council, the Alzheimer's Society and the British Heart Foundation.

Attention deficit (ADHD)

It is thought that about 4% of the population have a form of diagnosable Attention Deficit Hyperactivity Disorder (ADHD) which is usually associated with people, often children, who can't concentrate, are hyperactive, can be aggressive, are difficult to manage or teach, perform poorly academically and are generally troublesome. There is a wide range of ADHD symptoms and although it can affect anyone it is often hereditary.

As more research is done in this area it is becoming clearer as to what is actually happening in the brain and why people with this condition are behaving in the way they do. Effectively it is a malfunction of the brain's attention system, a diffuse linkage of neurons that binds together areas controlling arousal, motivation, reward and movement.

Although there are many types of possible treatments and ways to help manage the condition, including medication and CBT, it is now known that in several ways exercise can be very effective.

Physical activity, exercise and sport can provide great benefits for people with ADHD for a variety of reasons. In particular it can give them a focus that they wouldn't otherwise have and they can channel any energy and aggression into something that is positive and productive. It is thought that as many as 10% of elite sportsmen and -women have ADHD, and for certain sports it can actually be an advantage. Perhaps the most famous sportsperson with ADHD is the most successful Olympic athlete of all time, the swimmer Michael Phelps.

In the UK, two good examples are the Commonwealth Judo Gold medallist, Ashley McKenzie, and the Olympic medallist in Gymnastics, Louis Smith. Ashley McKenzie was unable to control his hyperactivity despite taking medication and was expelled from several schools, spent time in a young offenders' institution, and was banned from judo three times, for a total of 10 months, for drinking and fighting. Yet in 2014 he became Commonwealth Champion and has explained how the sport of judo completely changed his life and has been the major factor in controlling his ADHD.

These examples can be used to show that an ADHD child does not have to be written off as a 'naughty' child who is the result of bad parenting. Rather, with support from others, the condition can be turned into a positive, where children and adults can be encouraged to focus on their area of competence, with the success that that brings.

Addictive behaviour

Exercise and physical activity can serve as an antidote and as a type of inoculation against addiction because exercise sparks dopamine production, rebuilds toxic damage to the brain, battles anxiety and depression, and enhances self-esteem.

A definition of addiction can be 'a compulsion that persists in spite of negative health and social consequences'. Scientists now consider addiction to be a chronic disease because it wires in a memory that triggers reflexive behaviour. The same changes occur regardless of whether the addiction is to drugs or gambling or eating. Once the reward has the brain's attention, the prefrontal cortex instructs the hippocampus to remember the scenario and sensation in vivid detail.

Typically, when we learn something, the connections stabilise and the levels of dopamine tail off over time. With addiction, especially drug addiction, dopamine floods the system with each drug use, reinforcing the memory and pushing other stimuli further into the background.

If you suddenly quit drinking, for instance, you're turning off the dopamine spigot and the hypothalamic–pituitary–adrenal axis gets thrown out of balance. Withdrawal puts the body in survival mode. The intense unpleasantness of withdrawal lasts for only a few days, but your system remains sensitive for much longer. If you're in this delicate state and come under further stress, your brain interprets the situation as an emergency and sends you looking for more alcohol. That's how a problem at work or a fight with a lover can cause a relapse. For someone who's been dependent on drugs and has altered his dopamine system, the most effective solution to a stressful situation – and the only one he knows – is, unfortunately, the drug.

But exercise is another solution because it elevates the dopamine, which then improves mood, motivation, attention and feelings of wellness. Most exercise increases dopamine storage in the brain and triggers the production of enzymes that create dopamine receptors in the reward centre of the brain. If the demand is there, the dopamine genes are activated to produce more, and the overall effect is a more stable regulation of these pathways, which are important in controlling addictions.

Dealing with addiction is similar to battling feelings of anxiety and depression: getting rid of the problem is only the first step. Once the addiction or the negative emotions are gone, the void needs to be filled with some positive behaviour for the change to take root. There can hardly be a better option than physical exercise.

Exercise counteracts anxiety and depression directly and can have a huge impact on any form of addiction, as both of these mood states undermine treatment. A recovering addict who is feeling anxious or hopeless is much more likely to slip in her determination and ability to quit. People are more impulsive when they feel lousy.

Exercise also builds confidence. If the brain is flexible, the mind is stronger; a concept known as self-efficacy. It's difficult to measure, but it relates to confidence in our ability to change ourselves.

Most addicts, if they stop to consider how they may be destroying their life, suddenly feel like they can't handle anything, let alone maintain self-control over their addiction. Exercise, though, can have a powerful impact on the way an addict feels about himself. If he's engaged in a new pursuit such as exercise, which involves work and commitment, and he's able to follow through and be persistent with it, that sense of self- control spreads to other areas of his life.

As a treatment for addiction, exercise works from the top down in the brain, forcing addicts to adapt to a new stimulus and thereby allowing them to learn and appreciate alternative and healthy scenarios. It's activity-dependent training, and while it may not provide the immediate rush of a snort of cocaine, it instals a more diffuse sense of wellbeing that, over time, will become a craving in its own right. The inoculation against addiction works from the bottom up, physically blunting the urge to act by engaging the more primitive elements of the brain. Exercise builds synaptic detours around the well-worn connections automatically looking for the next fix.

Runner's high!

Many people would have heard of the expression 'runner's high' and the release of happy hormones called endorphins related to exercise and physical activity. Endorphins are chemicals that are able to cross through the gaps between neurons in order to pass along a message from one to the next. There are many different kinds, and much remains to be learned about their different purposes and functions.

One thing is known for certain about endorphins: their ability to make you feel oh-so-good. When your body is subjected to certain stimuli like sex, food or pain, your hypo-thalamus calls for endorphins, and the cells throughout your body that contain them heed the call. When endorphins lock into special receptor cells (called opioid receptors), they block the transmission of pain signals and also produce a euphoric feeling – exactly like opiates.

Endorphins act as both a painkiller and as the pay-off for your body's reward system.

When you hurt yourself (or eat a hot chilli pepper), you may get a big dose of endorphins to ease the pain. You may also get an endorphin blast from talking to a stranger, eating a satisfying meal or being exposed to ultraviolet light. (Everyone has different amounts of endorphins, and what may trigger an endorphin rush for one person could very well produce a dud for someone else.) The pay-off in the form of your body tapping into its own stash of 'opiates' is to let you know you've had enough – and convince you to do it again sometime soon.

Exercise stimulates endorphin production as well, but for a different reason, and it is often given the term 'runner's high', which refers to the euphoric feeling one sometimes gets when exercising. Researchers have found that light-to-moderate weight training or cardiovascular exercise doesn't produce endorphins, only heavy weights or training that incorporates sprinting or other anaerobic exertion.

When your body crosses over from an aerobic state to an anaerobic state, it's suddenly operating without enough oxygen to satisfy the muscles and cells screaming out for it. This is when the 'runner's high' occurs.

'Only exercise on the days you want to feel happy!'

Behavioural benefits

Doing more exercise, being more active and participating in more sports can have a very positive and beneficial effect on our overall behaviour. Exercise itself is positive and productive and below there are a number of more specific benefits that can result:

More energy, so more productive

Despite lack of energy and feeling too tired is often a reason for people not to exercise, the fact is that by doing more exercise you will increase your energy levels and feel less tired. With increased energy there are a number of direct benefits but in general it means you will be more productive. You will get more things done, achieve more and be more fulfilled as well as being less grumpy and grouchy because of the tiredness.

It may take a bit of time for your body to adjust and you may get some aching muscles or initially feel tired after exercising, but very soon your body will adapt and you will definitely feel more energised and therefore become more productive.

Social interaction

By doing more exercise and participating in physical activities it is more likely you will become more social through meeting new people, going to new places and trying new things out. You may join a club, a group or a team. You are likely to make new friends, which opens up other opportunities to be more social and do more things that you enjoy.

People of all ages and backgrounds can benefit at any time of their life, whether that's children playing together or older, retired people meeting up and enjoying social recreation. Generally the more social interaction people have the more they develop personally, with increased empathy and social skills, which are beneficial in all aspects of life.

Even if all your exercise and activities are done alone it will increase your confidence and give you more energy to do other things, so indirectly you are likely to become more sociable. Humans by nature are social creatures so this can only be a good thing, rather than finding yourself being or becoming quite reclusive.

Competitiveness

For a lot of people competition and feeling competitive is appealing and also beneficial, yet very often the opportunities to bring out this competitive spirit are few and far between in modern life. How often do you get the chance to be competitive in a physical or sporting way? For many of us there is an instinctive competitive element that is often subdued as there are not the opportunities to bring this out. However, many forms of exercise and activity can provide that sought-after competitiveness.

It could be a one-on-one sporting match, a team event, a larger running event or even setting your own personal goals to try and beat. All of these can provide healthy competition, which can provide a range of benefits.

Self-worth and pride

Whether or not you consciously recognise it, you will know that doing exercise or any physical activity is good for you and with that you can feel a sense of pride and self-worth that should not be underestimated. Feeling good about yourself is a wonderful thing and exercise and activities can provide that.

Whatever the activity you can feel pleased with yourself that you have done it. There may be lots of other reasons and benefits for doing the exercise but boosting your self-worth and pride is definitely one very positive effect. You have done something that most people don't do. You have done something that is good for you, for your health and for your happiness and this in turn can have many knock-on benefits, so try to recognise this very important element and give yourself a big pat on the back!

Achievement and fulfilment

It is very important for humans to have a purpose, be fulfilled and achieve things for a variety of reasons. Exercise and taking part in physical activities can be a great way of feeling fulfilled and it can provide you with that fantastic sense of achievement. No matter what the activity is, whether it's a thirty-minute walk or running a marathon, you have achieved something and should have that fulfilment and satisfaction feeling.

The more you do the more likely you are to want to do even more and perhaps set yourself some goals and challenges where you can achieve more and be even more fulfilled. That could be on an individual basis, with a partner or as part of a team. There are so many options and opportunities with exercise and activities that can give you that achievement and fulfilment.

Commitment and focus

The more involved you are in physical activity and exercise is the more likely it is that you will become more committed to it as you reap the benefits in a variety of ways. Feeling fitter and healthier, looking better, being more energised, meeting new people, increased confidence and self-esteem and improved mood are all likely benefits. And if this is happening it is more likely you will want more or at least not want to lose these benefits, so you will become more committed.

Having commitment is generally a very good quality and a positive behaviour which can knock on in a good way to other aspects of your life. You want to achieve something and you commit yourself to training or plans in order to be successful. You sign up to an exercise class, agree to run with a friend, enter a race or tournament, go on that activity holiday with a group, etc., which will all be positive and beneficial.

You are likely also to alter other behaviours in a good way such as getting more sleep, cutting down on the alcohol and eating a healthier diet, as well as thinking about upcoming activities and planning future exercise. You are likely to meet new people and seek out new opportunities in a positive way.

Whether you realise it or not you are likely to find yourself more committed to improving your health and happiness and having a very productive and positive focus. This focus will enable you to do more exercise, reduce or eliminate old excuses, be more productive generally and get more out of life, as well as be healthier and happier.

Positive attitude

In addition to being more committed and having an improved focus your attitude generally is likely to be much more positive. You will see and feel the results providing proof that doing more exercise is beneficial and that you can do it. There will be a sense of achievement aligned to all these other benefits, which in turn provides further desire to continue.

Your stress will reduce and your mood improve, making you a happier and more positive person to be around, and this will show. You are likely to get more compliments, have more to chat about to others and an increased belief in your abilities. So not only will you feel better in yourself you are likely to make others feel better and act as a motivator and inspiration to them.

A positive attitude is much more likely to attract more positivity than not and allows you and others around you to maintain and build upon those thoughts and behaviours. The enthusiasm generated can be infectious and the results hugely beneficial.

Looking forward

With a new positive outlook you will spend much more time looking forward than back, planning and preparing for future activities with a smile and enthusiasm. You will feel more alive, more confident and be better at dealing with the inevitable pieces of bad news and knocks that life brings.

You will spend much less time worrying about problems and issues that may exist in your life and much more time thinking about future activities and plans you have made. You are likely to feel more relaxed and contented with the new forward-looking, positive outlook. All of this will have additional benefits in many areas, which in turn will help you to continue improving your life in this way. Look forward with optimism, enthusiasm and energy rather than looking back with worry, regret and negativity.

Improved sleep

There is a common phrase that is often said to people after they have done a lot of exercise or activity, which is 'you will sleep well tonight'! And most people recognise that there is a relationship here between exercise and activity and then sleeping better as a result. There is much evidence to suggest that you will have better quality sleep if you have 'worn yourself out' as the body repairs, replenishes, rests and recovers.

It may not be possible or practical to 'wear yourself out' each day through exercise and activities but bear in mind that exercise will help you sleep and improve its quality. So if you have sleep issues here is another great reason to exercise.

The importance of sleep for mental wellbeing was highlighted in a recent report by the Mental Health Foundation. This report also highlighted that up to one-third of the population may suffer from insomnia (lack of sleep or poor-quality sleep). Insomnia can negatively affect mood, energy and concentration levels, relationships, and people's ability to stay awake and function during the day. Physical activity may enhance sleep quality, which in turn improves wellbeing. A recent survey collected objective physical activity data and responses to questions on sleep from 3081 adults and found that higher levels of physical activity were associated with fewer reports of feeling overly sleepy during the day and less difficulty concentrating when tired.

Research with people who have long-term difficulties with initiating and maintaining sleep (chronic primary insomnia) has found physical activity can be used as an intervention to enhance sleep quality and improve quality of life. A single session of 50 minutes' moderate intensity aerobic exercise was found to reduce pre-sleep anxiety and improve sleep in patients with chronic primary insomnia. A six-month physical activity intervention (50 minutes moderate intensity exercise, 3 times per week) resulted in improved sleep, greater quality of life and reduced negative moods such as tension, depression and anger.

Improved nutrition

There is often a correlation between what you eat and drink and the exercise and activities you do. If you get into a pattern where you do very little exercise you may well have a poor diet, too, so you struggle for energy, become more lethargic, have a lower mood and find yourself eating more snacks or high sugar- and carbohydrate-content food, as well as perhaps comfort eating more. On the other hand, if you are doing more exercise and activities you may find yourself eating an improved, more balanced, more nutritional diet and probably drinking less alcohol too.

Many people will comfort eat and use food and drink to try and make them feel better or as a reaction to something that has happened. Usually these foods are very unhealthy and although they may provide a short-term fix for our mood, they soon have the opposite effect and can have several consequences like weight gain and feeling more lethargic, with lower confidence and self-esteem. Some people will have eating issues and disorders whereby they don't eat enough; exercising can stimulate appetite and help someone to eat and drink a healthy diet and put on weight if that is the healthier objective.

Of course, this isn't always the case, but as a generalisation people do tend to improve their food intake and eat and drink more healthily in conjunction with a healthy physical activity and exercise programme, which leads to an even better all round lifestyle.

'Let exercise be your stress reliever... not food.'

Physical health benefits

'Those who think they have no time for exercise will sooner or later have to find time for illness.'

Obesity and weight problems

For many people one of the main reasons for exercising is to lose weight or to maintain their weight, and everyone is aware that being physically active and doing exercise can help in this way. The most obvious direct way that exercise helps with weight is through burning calories. Generally the more active you are and the more exercise you do the more calories you burn off.

The simplest equation for weight loss is to burn off more calories than you consume, and this is usually done and most effective with a combination of exercise and calorie consumption (i.e. food and drink intake). Your metabolism also plays a role and exercise can increase or boost your metabolism, which means you burn calories at a higher rate and for longer. So exercise doesn't just help burn calories when you are active, it can help you burn more for several hours afterwards, too.

Many people who are overweight may feel too unfit to exercise and there can be some risks involved in participating in physical activity. However, your body is very good at adjusting and adapting so as long as you are sensible, and build up slowly and steadily; then your body will get used to the exercise and you will be able to do much more. And the more you do the more likely you are to benefit and lose weight effectively.

Your confidence, self-esteem and mood are all likely to improve, which will provide further motivation to be more active and continue to lose weight and be physically healthier. Obesity can lead to many direct and indirect health problems and exercise is a safe, effective and convenient way to lose weight and improve health. You might even enjoy it and find some hidden talents. There are many examples of obese people who have taken up running or cycling and have not only gone on to lose significant weight but have become very good athletes and now participate in competitive sport!

Cleansing the body

Many of the real benefits of exercise are hidden beneath the surface, and it appears that one of these is the fact that exercise can speed up the removal of 'rubbish' from inside our body's cells; exercise helps the cells sweep away unwanted debris like viruses and bacteria that infect us or build up over time.

It also helps prevent or treat constipation, helping to maintain regular bowel movements. Most forms of activity and exercise will be beneficial if you exert enough effort to break sweat, which is also a great cleanser. Sweat is really good for your skin and helps push out the bad toxins and unwanted debris you accumulate. So, effectively, exercise is a great detoxifier and helps to cleanse our bodies.

Included in this is the brain, and the positive cleansing effect exercise can have on this vital organ could help prevent conditions like dementia as well as helping to maintain our memory, alertness, concentration and coordination.

Heart and lungs

Many studies have shown the clear benefits of physical activity for your heart and lungs. When done regularly, moderate- and vigorous-intensity physical activity strengthens your heart muscle. This improves your heart's ability to pump blood to your lungs and throughout your body. As a result, more blood flows to your muscles, and oxygen levels in your blood rise. Capillaries, your body's tiny blood vessels, also widen, allowing them to deliver more oxygen to your body and carry away waste products.

When done regularly, moderate- and vigorous-intensity aerobic activity can lower your risk for CHD. This is a condition in which a waxy substance called plaque builds up inside your coronary arteries. These arteries supply your heart muscle with oxygen-rich blood; plaque narrows the arteries and reduces blood flow to your heart muscle. Eventually, an area of plaque can rupture (break open), causing a blood clot to form on the surface of the plaque. If the clot becomes large enough, it can mostly or completely block blood flow through a coronary artery. Blocked blood flow to the heart muscle causes a heart attack.

Inactive people are nearly twice as likely to develop CHD as people who are physically active. Studies suggest that inactivity is a major risk factor for CHD, just like high blood pressure, high blood cholesterol, and smoking. For people who have CHD, aerobic activity done regularly helps the heart work better. It also may reduce the risk of a second heart attack in people who have already had heart attacks.

With more exercise you are likely to increase your oxygen capacity, not be so breathless, be more in control of your breathing and generally feel fitter. Your body will be more efficient, you will feel stronger, reduce your risk of several diseases and conditions mentioned and will be able to do much more with your life, which is likely to be a longer one.

Blood pressure

High blood pressure is known as hypertension and is commonly referred to as the 'silent killer' because it usually has very few obvious symptoms yet can be fatal. Around 30% of people in the UK have high blood pressure but many don't know it; if left untreated, high blood pressure increases your risk of a heart attack or stroke. The only real way of knowing if there is a problem is to have your blood pressure measured regularly.

As you get older your blood pressure tends to rise naturally, which increases your risk of health issues; however, exercise has been proven to be very effective in maintaining and indeed lowering blood pressure levels. Being more active and taking regular exercise lowers blood pressure by keeping your heart and blood vessels in good condition. Regular exercise can also help you lose weight, which will also help lower your blood pressure.

Diabetes

In the UK there are now over 3 million people or 6% of the population diagnosed with diabetes and this figure is growing at an alarming rate. It does not include all those people who have diabetes but have not been diagnosed. There are two types of diabetes (1 and 2), and it is type 2 that is by far the most common (around 90%) and also the one most associated with lifestyle factors.

Diabetes can cause serious long-term health problems. It's the most common cause of visual impairment and blindness in people of working age. It's also responsible for most cases of kidney failure and lower limb amputation (other than accidents). People with diabetes are up to five times more likely to have cardiovascular disease and stroke than those without diabetes.

Physical activity can help prevent or delay the onset of type 2 diabetes. It is particularly effective in the prevention of type 2 diabetes in people who are sedentary. Physical activity appears to be the strongest predictor in reducing the incidence of type 2 diabetes in the absence of any change in weight, blood pressure or cholesterol.

People who have diabetes are encouraged to exercise regularly for better blood-sugar control and to reduce the risk of cardiovascular diseases. The reason for this is that muscles which are working use more glucose than those that are resting, and the more muscle you have, the more excess blood sugar it can store. Muscle movement leads to greater sugar uptake by muscle cells and lower blood-sugar levels.

Any form of physical activity and exercise will be beneficial in preventing diabetes and helping to manage and improve the condition. If you feel tired much of the time, are often thirsty, are overweight and do little exercise you should see your doctor and get tested for diabetes.

Cholesterol

There are two types of cholesterol – low-density lipoprotein (LDL) and high-density lipoprotein (HDL) cholesterol. LDL cholesterol is often called 'bad' cholesterol whilst HDL cholesterol is often called 'good' cholesterol. High levels of LDL and low levels of HDL increase your risk of heart disease, heart attacks and strokes. High cholesterol itself does not cause any symptoms so getting your levels checked and monitored is important, especially if your lifestyle suggests you are at risk.

You can help to improve the balance of your cholesterol through physical activity, though. Exercise helps improve your cholesterol levels indirectly in many ways such as lowering blood pressure and reducing your weight. However, being active and taking regular exercise will directly help to increase the levels of 'good cholesterol' (HDL) in your body by stimulating the body to move fatty deposits to the liver so they can be broken down.

Cancers

There is lots of evidence that being more physically active can reduce the risk of developing some types of cancer. Scientists have developed some good theories for how this might work. It's likely that different effects are important in different types of cancer.

Hormones are chemical messengers that get carried around our bodies in our blood; they help tell our bodies and cells what to do. Being physically active can change the levels of some hormones, including oestrogen and insulin. In women physical activity can lower the level of oestrogen. Oestrogen is thought to fuel the development of many breast and womb cancers, so reducing the levels of this hormone could help to reduce the risk.

Activity can also reduce the amount of insulin in our blood. Insulin is very important in controlling how our bodies use and store energy from food. Changes in insulin levels can have effects all over the body. And scientists think insulin can turn on signals that tell cells to multiply. Because cancer starts when cells multiply out of control, lowering insulin levels could help stop some types of cancer developing.

Helping food to move through our bowel more quickly reduces the amount of time that the lining of the bowel is in contact with any harmful chemicals, like those related to alcohol, and red and processed meat. So there's less chance of them being able to do any damage that could lead to cancer.

Inflammation is a normal part of the way our bodies react to injury or infections, but it can sometimes cause even more damage, particularly when it keeps happening in the same place. This can lead to the cells multiplying much more frequently than usual, to replace dead and damaged cells, which means there is more chance of the mistakes that can lead to cancer. Being physically active helps to keep inflammation under control in our bowel, reducing the risk of cancer developing.

Additionally, for many people who have cancer and are going through treatment it is important for lots of reasons to maintain regular physical activity and exercise if possible. The exercise could directly help with the cancer but also will help in other areas that provide a better quality of life during this period.

Jane Tomlinson continued with exercise and indeed set herself many more physical challenges after she had been diagnosed with terminal cancer. Not only did she insist she lived many more years longer as a result, she was able to do so many positive things and lead a much more fulfilling and rewarding life during this time as a result of her exercise and challenges. Plus she raised millions for charity, as well as inspiring so many other people in the process.

Bones, muscles and joints

One in three people in the UK have lower back pain each year, but people who exercise are less likely to get it. If you have lower back pain, exercise can often help to reduce it and also prevent further or future issues. Building up your core strength can be done in a number of ways, including yoga and Pilates as well as weightlifting, circuit training, swimming and running.

Moderate activity, including walking, swimming and cycling, can also help to treat and reduce pain caused by osteoarthritis. This is a common form of arthritis, with about 8.5 million people in the UK affected by the condition.

Physical activity in younger people and children can increase bone mineral density and help to maintain strong bones. It also slows down bone degeneration later in life. Regular exercise can help to prevent osteoporosis – when your bones become brittle and more prone to breaking. But if you already have osteoporosis, it's better to choose weight-bearing exercise, such as walking or dancing.

Joints require motion to stay healthy, and long periods of inactivity cause the arthritic joint to stiffen and the adjoining tissue to weaken. Your muscles need blood and oxygen to remove cellular waste and produce energy for physical activity. Exercising improves your muscular system with repetitive muscle contractions, such as flexing your legs while walking on the treadmill or flexing your arms while lifting weights. The blood and oxygen flowing into your muscles increases and decreases, so the exercise improves your muscular system by improving circulation and enhances the energy and waste-removal capacity in your muscle tissues.

Muscular endurance is required for flexing your muscles repeatedly, and for sustaining muscular contractions against resistance for extended periods of time. Exercise, particularly high-repetition weightlifting, can increase this muscular endurance. Greater muscular endurance can improve your quality of life. For example, core muscle endurance helps you maintain a healthy posture, which optimises the flow of nutrients throughout your body.

Exercise can improve your muscular system by increasing your muscle strength. Resistance exercise, such as weightlifting, is the ideal form of exercise for strength training. A stronger muscular system can generate more force against resistance, and allows you to move heavier weight over greater distances. The diameter of your muscles expands as they get stronger, which protects your bones and joints from problems such as osteoporosis and arthritis.

Maintaining your balance while performing complex joint movements requires muscular coordination. Athletic training involves exercises that improve coordination for sports-specific skills. Daily activities such as showering, unloading groceries and household chores all require muscular coordination. Exercise helps you maintain and improve coordination by forming neuromuscular pathways which allow your muscular system to communicate with your nervous and other bodily systems more effectively. Walking, balance-board training and weightlifting with free weights help your muscular system coordinate joint movements more effectively.

Hair and skin

By increasing blood flow, exercise helps nourish skin cells and keep them healthy. In addition to providing oxygen, blood flow also helps carry away waste products, including free radicals, from working cells. The job of neutralising toxins belongs mostly to the liver, but by increasing blood flow a bout of exercise helps flush cellular debris out of the system.

Exercise has also been shown to ease stress, and by decreasing stress, some conditions that can be exacerbated by stress can show some improvement. These include acne and eczema. Although researchers are still investigating the link between stress and skin, studies show that the sebaceous glands, which produce oil in the skin, are influenced by stress hormones.

As exercise helps increase blood flow this also applies to the scalp, enabling the release of nutrients into the hair follicles, which stimulates growth and releases toxins. Rigorous exercise can help you work up a good sweat, and since toxins are released through sweat, this works as a cleansing regimen for the skin and scalp, which in turn creates a healthy environment for hair to grow. So regular exercise that makes you sweat can be just as effective or maybe even better than all the expensive moisturisers, lotions, shampoos and conditioners!

Ageing

Getting wrinkles are an inevitable part of ageing, but scientists have revealed that you may be able to maintain your skin's youth without pumping it full of chemicals or spending vast sums of money. New research has found that exercise may not only keep skin younger, it may also even reverse skin ageing in people who become more active late in life.

Exercise does far more than just keep your body in good order – it can actually turn back the clock. More and more research shows that working out can help your brain, bones, heart and skin look and act younger. 'The secret to anti-ageing isn't about creams and lotions, but about how to build a foundation from the inside-out with a strong body and a sound mind,' says Kathy Smith, spokesperson for the International Council on Active Ageing.

Increasing blood flow to any area of the body promotes the metabolism in that area, and it makes sense that when you exercise toxins will get flushed out and cells will heal and grow faster. In other words, more blood to your dermis provides a better environment for collagen growth and promotes younger-looking skin.

Independence in old age

There is no question that overall people are living longer and this is likely to continue indefinitely. Of course, that is generally seen as a good thing, though quality of life is very important and exercise and physical activity can play a very positive role in improving this as people get older.

If you have done exercise and continue to do so then your body will be stronger and more flexible. Your bones and joints are more likely to be in decent shape and your breathing will be better. You will be more agile and your balance and coordination will deteriorate less. This all means that you are likely to be more independent and less reliant on others. Additionally your risk of falling, breaking bones and causing other injuries will be much reduced and your sex life is likely to be extended.

You will be able to lead a more active and participative life than if you were sedentary. You can be more sociable and do more things with your life and therefore continue to live a much richer and rewarding life for longer. Having that greater independence and improved health will certainly improve your quality of life and also that of those around you. So exercise and physical activity is important at all ages, and the longer you can maintain this the better your life will be.

Hormonal issues and menopause

Hormone imbalances can occur in men and women of almost any age. A variety of factors can be related to these imbalances, including high insulin levels from diets high in refined foods and sugar, exposure to environmental toxins (xenoestrogens), high consumption of hydrogenated fats, and lack of physical activity leading to weight gain.

Age is also a factor in reduced levels of hormones, creating feelings of imbalance in everyday pursuits. For example, testosterone levels in women begin going down after age 20. By age 40 a woman's testosterone level will be half of what it was when she was 20 years old. This is why getting hormone levels checked even while in your 20s may be necessary if you aren't feeling yourself. For women between the ages of 40 and 60, testosterone levels can remain pretty constant. After menopause testosterone declines once again.

Physical activity is important to hormone balance, not to mention overall health and a good mental state. Cortisol levels can become significantly high when the body is experiencing stress, either real or imagined. Exercise helps counter the effects of stress and regular moderate exercise can lower cortisol levels. Moderate exercise for 30 to 60 minutes each day can have a profound effect on hormone balance.

There's evidence that women who do regular exercise and are generally more active tend to suffer less from the symptoms of the menopause.

Menopausal symptoms can include:

- hot flushes and night sweats
- loss of libido (sex drive)
- vaginal dryness and pain, itching or discomfort during sex
- palpitations (heartbeats that suddenly become more noticeable)
- headaches
- mood changes, such as depression, anxiety or tiredness
- sleeping problems, such as insomnia
- urinary tract infections (UTIs)

Smoking and other drugs

People who exercise regularly and are physically active tend to smoke less and take fewer drugs. There are many reasons for this but one of the factors is the fact that exercise itself can work like a drug. Chemicals are released within the brain and the body that can provide similar effects to the 'highs' you may get with drugs and smoking, and so people can get a 'fix' through physical activity, which is much healthier. We all know the serious health risks and damage that smoking and other drugs can do to us.

In addition exercise can lower stress, anxiety and depression, which can often be linked to smoking and drug taking. It can boost confidence and self-esteem, and many of the reasons why people smoke and take drugs are reduced by participating in exercise. Boredom is another factor and by exercising, being more active or doing sports this can be reduced, too.

You will also find that in a healthier, sporty, exercise- and activity-motivated environment fewer people will smoke or take drugs, so there is less influence or peer pressure and indeed there is far more expectation and encouragement not to smoke or take drugs, which in turn becomes a greater incentive and motivation not to smoke, or at least to cut down. And finally, if you want to improve your fitness, are setting new goals, are challenging yourself and want to be healthier, then a more active lifestyle with more exercise is going to make you want to smoke a lot less or quit altogether.

Alcohol

Generally speaking, the more active you are and the more exercise and sport you participate in then the less alcohol you will drink. Of course there are exceptions and some sports and social activities may in fact encourage more drinking. However, if you look at many of the reasons why people drink alcohol then it makes a lot of sense that in general less alcohol will be consumed.

Some of the reasons why people drink, and drink more than is recommended, include boredom, stress, anxiety, depression, not being able to sleep, lack of focus and commitment and little emphasis on personal health. Exercise and physical activity can help and be beneficial in all those areas.

Exercise can relieve boredom and give people a focus where they are more committed. It can help manage, treat and prevent stress, anxiety and depression and it can help you sleep better too. Plus a more health-conscious lifestyle including exercise is likely to highlight alcohol as a potential problem and therefore you are more likely to drink less.

Finally, if any alcohol issue is more of an addiction then we have already seen that exercise can be very beneficial for addictions and addictive behaviour through the regulation and uplift of certain neurotransmitters, including dopamine.

Employers

On average individuals spend a third of their waking time and over 40 years of their lives at work. The increasingly sedentary nature of work means that for many people much of this time is spent being physically inactive. Evidence is accumulating to show that it is cost-effective for employers to promote employee physical activity, as this has a range of positive outcomes for employees themselves and knock-on business benefits. For example, physically active employees take on average 27% fewer sick days, are less likely to suffer from major health problems, and less likely to have an accident at work.

Physically active employees have also been shown to have lower levels of presenteeism; this is when employees are at work but not fully engaged or productive. Physically active employees tend to have greater job satisfaction, greater mental alertness and greater self-confidence.

Indirect benefits have also been reported, such as enhanced company reputation and improved team working. Workplace physical activity interventions can encourage physical activity by providing opportunities to be active during the work day. Examples here include encouraging employees to use the stairs rather than the lift (posters stating the wellbeing benefits of stair-walking placed at the lift doors can be effective prompts), or scheduling an appointment to meet a colleague for a walk rather than in a meeting room and have the meeting whilst walking. Clearly this would not be suitable for all meetings but it can be surprisingly productive.

Employers can also encourage employees to be active during their breaks and before and after work. For example, many employers provide an on-site gym or discount at a local leisure facility, or offer employees reductions on the cost of bicycles through the government's Cycle to Work scheme. Setting up lunchtime walking groups, a group pedometer challenge, or other group activities such as yoga can also increase activity levels. It has been shown that nominating one or two workplace Physical Activity Champion(s) can be an effective way of encouraging staff to take up and maintain the exercise and activities. These individuals take on the role of motivating other employees to be active, act as a local source of information about physical activity opportunities, and help to create social networks around physical activity in the workplace.

Environmental changes such as providing safe bicycle storage and shower and changing facilities can support employees to take up physical activity. An important contributing factor to the success of workplace physical activity programmes is management support, as this helps to create a workplace culture which is supportive of physical activity.

Part 3

Exercise and Activity Options

Types of exercise

There is such a huge range of physical activity that can be classed as exercise and there really is something for everyone. Take time to think about all the different potential exercise options there are and how they could become part of your life, or at least whether you are willing to try them out.

Here are some examples of different types of exercise and I am sure you can think of some more!

Walking, Hiking, Running, Climbing, Swimming, Cycling, Pilates, Yoga, Dancing, Aerobics, Zumba, Martial Arts, Football, Rugby, Cricket, Tennis, Squash, Badminton, Softball, Lacrosse, Hockey, Netball, Basketball, Golf, Athletics, Circuit training, Horse riding, Sailing, Rowing, Skating, Skiing, Sex, Weightlifting, Gymnastics, Bowling, Gardening, Housework and many more!

What do you enjoy or did you used to enjoy?

There are so many options when it comes to exercise and activities that it is worth taking time to really think about what you want to do, why you want to do it and how you will do it. Think about any activities you have previously done and enjoyed. Can you do this again? Why did you enjoy it? Think about it in a positive way and make plans to take it up again.

Are you able to do more of the activities you enjoy? Perhaps you can do them more regularly or with different groups or in different places? Chat to friends, family members and work colleagues about what they do or would like to do and see if anything grabs your interest and enthusiasm.

The more you enjoy something the more likely you are to do it, to make the effort and to stick with it. So if you know you enjoy something then start with that, but if you can't think of anything or there are limited options then think carefully about all the other possibilities and give some a try. You won't know whether you like it or not until you try, and the more options you have the better.

Recently I started going to 'Street Dance' classes, which are great fun and also a great workout. I do a lot of exercise and activities already, but I was thinking about what else I could do or try that might be of interest and my mind turned to dancing. I have never danced before except when I was a lot younger, at discos and clubs and usually after several drinks, though I did used to enjoy dancing on these occasions. So, enjoying music and the idea of dancing I quickly came across a local group after mentioning the idea to a friend – it has been great, and something I will continue with. It uses a few different muscle groups to my usual activities, it is a lot of fun and burns lots of calories, with a great bunch of people.

'Never underestimate the power of passion.' – Eve Sawyer

What would you like to try?

Life should be enjoyable, you should try and do things that make you smile, that you want to do and that are good for you as much as possible and practical. Life is also about living and not just existing, so it is important to try things and find out what you like and don't like. When it comes to exercise, sport and physical activities there are so many possibilities and things you could try.

So think about what you would like to try if you could. Take away all the potential barriers like being scared, not knowing how to do something, not having the money, not having the time or having nobody to try it with. What does the list look like if there are no barriers?

Now think about how good it is not to have regrets, to step out of your comfort zone every now and then, to scare yourself from time to time and to really feel alive. Think about investing money in your health and happiness rather than just the cost of something and think about investing time into your life for these activities, because the rewards are more than worth it.

It may be something completely new or an activity that requires a lot of skill to learn and if so then be patient and build up slowly over time. Believe that you can do it and the time and dedication will be rewarded.

Try researching on the internet for the opportunities, people, groups, organisations and clubs that may be helpful in your quest. Speak to friends, family and colleagues for ideas, advice, encouragement and motivation, and try those things that appeal to you. If you start doing activities that are enjoyable, fun, rewarding and healthy then that is a fantastic place to be and to continue with. If you find a passion, make new friends, become fitter and healthier, increase your confidence and everything else those activities can bring then you will be so much happier and really living your life. So go for it!

Gyms, groups, clubs, boot camps and sports clubs

Most people will have access to a wide range of exercise, sporting and physical activity opportunities close to where they live, which can be very beneficial. Although factors such as cost, equipment, timings, work patterns and family life practicalities may all have to be taken into account, there is usually something for everybody if you look into the options.

Gyms and health clubs are very common and although they can vary in types of membership, facilities, costs and opening times there are often many choices including pay as you go, off-peak membership, 24-hour access and special deals throughout the year. Gyms and health clubs can provide an excellent environment in which to train, attend classes, meet new people, go with friends or family, go on your own, get expert advice and guidance, get free inductions and much more.

Outdoor boot camps have become increasingly popular in recent years and most towns and cities will have a wide range of options for all abilities. Being outdoors in the fresh air with a range of exercises and other people can be a fun, enjoyable and social experience as well as being a great form of exercise.

There are also many clubs you can join or go along to in a wide range of activities and a variety of different sports including running, hiking, sailing, rowing, martial arts, dance, keep fit, etc. Often they are very low-cost and sometimes free. Again they can be social and fun, and cater for a wide range of abilities. Talk to friends and work colleagues about what they know or do a quick internet search and you will undoubtedly find many options available.

All these opportunities are there for you and can provide huge benefits if you participate, invest your time and commit to them. You have nothing to lose and so much to gain in so many ways!

Events and challenges

Have you ever participated in a big physical activity event of any kind? Whether it be a 5k race, a half-marathon or full marathon, a cycling race, a swimming gala, an organised charity walk, an outdoor obstacle course, a charity mountain climb or anything that combines exercise with lots of people?

If you have you know how great they can be! The atmosphere, the excitement, the nerves, the camaraderie, the encouragement, the support and the sense of achievement and pride they can produce. If not then you have missed out and I would encourage you to try it. Apart from all the benefits you get from training for the event, you can benefit so much more from the experience and your achievement.

Have a think about what you could do or would want to try and aim for. Even if you have never done anything before it is possible for nearly everyone to run a 5-kilometre race with a few months' training, if you build up slowly and sensibly. Plus it's not about the winning or the times, it is about the participation, the experience and the achievement. There is also the opportunity to do it for a good cause too, which is likely to further enhance your experience and achievement by gaining extra support and encouragement and by helping others in the process.

Stop sitting

The act of sitting can literally make your bum bigger! Research found through using MRI scans of muscle tissue that sitting around for long periods of time could put pressure on cells and cause the body to produce 50% more fat that it normally would do. It suggests that when force is applied to a specific area of the body for an extended time, it causes fat tissue to expand.

Also, as you sit down, the electrical activity in your leg muscles shuts off and the number of calories you burn falls significantly, plus enzyme production, which helps break down fat, drops by up to 90%. Additionally your good cholesterol levels drop and all these effects combined really have a very negative effect on your health. Even if you do a lot of other exercise you are at some danger if you sit around for long periods of time

Another reason for not sitting around for long periods is that your blood sugar and insulin levels will spike to potentially dangerous levels, but getting up and moving about regularly will counterbalance this.

So try sitting around for less time and take frequent breaks in which you get up and walk around for a minute or two. Get into the habit of sitting at your desk for no more than twenty minutes before some kind of initiated action. Stand up, move your legs, squat down or do a little jiggle! If you can break the habit of sitting for long periods of time it will make a big difference in many ways and you will soon get into a much better habit of being an 'active' sitter.

Stepometers and pedometers

A very simple yet very effective little device you can buy is a stepometer or pedometer-type gadget, which effectively measures how many steps you take over a period of time. They can be wristbands, watches, small clip-on devices or even necklaces. Once you start using one you can quickly find out how many 'steps' you do per day and then start setting particular targets to increase this.

For example, it may be that on average in your first week you do around 6,000 steps per day. However, if you set a target of 8,000 steps and are able to monitor it regularly you will find that you can fairly easily increase your activity to reach that new target. Then once you have reached this you can aim for even more, say 10,000 steps per day on average. This doesn't mean you have to do loads more exercise, because a few extra steps here and there, a slightly longer walk at lunchtime, a bit more moving around at work, etc., quickly add up to a lot more steps.

You can then get a rough idea of the extra calories burned, which will add up significantly to your weekly count. Having the monitor and setting targets is a great yet simple way to be more active and, of course, you can always have a competition with your partner, family member or friend to motivate you even more. Also, many of these devices have additional features and you are able to download all the information quickly and easily to help record your efforts.

A recent study showed that the average American only reached 5,117 steps per day whilst the average Australian reached a more impressive 9,695 steps per day, almost double the rate. This perhaps also helps explain why Australia's obesity rate is 16% whilst in the United States it is 34%.

Active at work and home

When you are awake you will most likely spend the vast majority of your time either at work or at home. If you think about how many hours per day this covers then there is a huge opportunity to be more active in these places, which could have significant benefits. Of course there are many practicalities that may restrict you but there will undoubtedly be things you can do to increase your activity levels and therefore improve your health.

Depending on your work environment and the obvious practicalities, think about how you can be more active. Walking up the stairs rather than using a lift, parking your car further away and walking, getting up from your desk and walking around the office regularly, going for a walk outside at lunchtime or other breaks, moving your legs under the desk, etc. Over the course of a week you could easily burn an additional 1,000 calories by just intentionally being a bit more active at work, making a big difference with hardly any real effort.

There could be some exercise classes, running clubs or walking groups already organised or you could help set some up. Chat to other people at work who may also want to increase their activity levels and see what options there are.

At home there are lots of exercises and activities you can do specifically as well as more generally. You could do some specific workouts at home, maybe using a DVD or music which could be either dancing, aerobic workouts, exercise bike, weights, yoga or weight-bearing exercises. These could be for as little as five minutes at a time to a full hour. There are lots of equipment pieces that could further aid your activities.

Then again it is more about intentionally being a little more active, by getting up from the sofa or chair more often, walking up and down the stairs more, waving your arms about (when no one is looking!), moving your legs up and down while sitting, etc. There is a lot you can do at home that increases your activity levels, burns calories, increases your fitness and in turn improves your health. Plus the more you do the easier it becomes and the longer term the benefits.

> *'Exercise doesn't get in the way of my life... It adds to the quality of my life.'*

Dealing with injuries

Although exercise and being physically active will improve strength and fitness and help to prevent injuries, there is still the risk that injuries can occur. You should never be put off exercise because of the possibility of getting injured; many potential injuries can be avoided by being sensible and not taking unnecessary risks. For example, making sure you wear the right clothing and footwear, warm up and cool down, stretch properly and build up slowly. Taking the right advice, listening to your body and not overtraining will also help to prevent injury.

However, if you do get injured then how you deal with it is important. There is a risk that you can make things worse, thus prolonging the injury and time out. You may also feel down as a result of being injured and not being able to exercise as you want, and you may put on weight as you burn considerably fewer calories. So firstly be aware of the potential downsides to injury, but then try to ensure you deal with them effectively.

Do your own research on the injury and try to understand what you have done, how best to recover and rehabilitate in the most effective way. It is worth seeing a specialist physiotherapist if you feel the injury is bad or do not know what it actually is. Investing some money on this expertise is likely to be worth it if the injury is bad. You will need to be patient, but see what other exercise and activities may be possible while you recover from the injury. For example you may be able to swim or cycle rather than run, or work on upper-body conditioning if you have a foot or leg injury.

If you cannot do any exercise for a period seek other things you can do that will help, like reading books, finding new hobbies or thinking about future goals and challenges to keep you motivated. Be careful of your diet and compensate by eating less if you are unable to be active. You may be disappointed, frustrated, annoyed and upset by your injury, but it is up to you how you deal with it and get through the recovery time in the best way.

Part 4

How to Get Motivated to Exercise

'If it is important to you, you will find a way. If not, you will find an excuse.'

Introduction

The formal dictionary definition of 'motivation' is *'a reason or reasons for acting or behaving in a particular way'*.

The psychological definition of 'motivation' is *'the process that initiates, guides and maintains goal-orientated behaviours. It involves the biological, emotional, social and cognitive forces that activate behaviour.'*

Motivation plays a huge role in our lives in so many ways and can often be the key factor in whether we do something or not and then whether we succeed in that objective or not. With regard to doing exercise and being physically active it is also a big factor. It would be so much easier and we would do so much more exercise if we were more motivated! So it is very important to try and understand all the reasons and factors personal to us as to why we are or are not motivated and the levels of motivation we have and can have.

I believe there are four key components of motivation, as follows:

The starting point – there has to be an initial starting point for your motivation, perhaps a goal or challenge you have thought of, or someone else has planted an idea that sparks an interest. From this initial point there comes the activation of the idea and you start to plan and prepare until you actually commit to that particular goal. The motivation is usually quite high in the initial stages with a burst of optimism and enthusiasm.

Endurance – this is how long you can maintain the effort, and your level of persistence. It will require endurance and stamina to remain motivated so that you can achieve the goal. Are you able to keep going, overcome any hurdles or setbacks and persist with your efforts?

Intensity of effort – then there is how committed you really are to the goal, how much effort and hard work you will dedicate to the challenge and how much you want it. Are you prepared to give it your best, to focus, to make sacrifices and to keep motivating yourself so that the goal is achieved?

The end goal – finally there is the reward and sense of achievement you get from completing the goal and challenge. By focusing on the end result and reminding yourself of the reasons for the challenge and the benefits of achieving your goals you will be better placed to maintain your motivation.

All four components are important in order to be successful. If any one of them is missing or neglected then you are more likely to struggle with your motivation and therefore less likely to achieve your goals.

'Do something today that your future self will thank you for!'

There is another book in this series entitled *Motivation, Achievement & Challenges*, which goes into much more depth about motivation. It discusses the reasons that can affect motivation as well as the wide range of factors that can increase and improve it, and provides some real-life motivational stories and practical tips. I would recommend reading the book as it will be both interesting and beneficial.

You can order a copy or download from Amazon or iTunes or go to the www.climbyourmountain.org website for more details.

'Be the change you want to see in the world' – *Mahatma Gandhi*

Challenge yourself

Have you ever really challenged yourself or been challenged? Have you ever pushed yourself to or been pushed to the limits? Have you ever found out what you are truly capable of doing, overcoming and achieving? The chances are you haven't. Most of us never have and never will push ourselves to the limits and really find out our true potential. That's OK, and most of the time there really is no need to do this. Also it can be very tough and very hard work plus a lot of pain and sacrifice.

However, if you do challenge yourself and push towards those limits you will find out what you really are capable of. What a great feeling once you have achieved or overcome something where it has required more than you thought you had, you gave more than you think you could give and you were much stronger than you ever thought you were. By challenging yourself you will find out so much more about yourself. Your strengths and weaknesses will become clearer, your confidence will rise, the real you will be exposed and your levels of pride will become even greater.

> *'Strength doesn't come from what you can do, it comes from overcoming the things you once thought you couldn't.'*

You will have inner strength and capabilities that you didn't realise you had if you push yourself. And once you realise you have those additional qualities and abilities it will provide you with greater confidence to go on to achieve more, challenge yourself further and overcome anything that life throws at you in the future. Don't be like most people who will never find out what they are capable of and what their true potential is. There is so much more you can do, can accomplish and can deal with when the situation requires it. So don't just wait until something challenges you, go and challenge yourself now. Go and see what you are capable of both physically and mentally and give it your best.

> *'The greatest danger for most of us is not that our aim is too high and we miss it, but that it is too low and we reach it.'* – Michelangelo

CYM trips and challenges

UK trips and challenges

In the UK, Climb Your Mountain (CYM) has been offering a range of trips and challenges since 2008 and below are some of the examples with a bit more detail about each one, what is involved and what typically happens. Anyone can participate in order to feel good, have a great time, achieve something special and support the charity. Safety is always the first priority, closely followed by making the experience as friendly and enjoyable as possible for all those who join us.

Snowdon

Snowdon is the highest mountain in Wales at 1,085m (3,560ft) and lies in the Snowdonia National Park in North Wales. It is the most common trip we do with CYM, usually about 10 weekend trips per year. There are several different routes up and down that we choose from depending on weather conditions, time of the year and the group participating. A typical weekend would be to travel up on Saturday morning and do a gentle walk of 2–3 hours in the afternoon somewhere in the area. There are a selection of fantastic, beautiful walks to choose from. We will then head to the hotel to relax and enjoy an evening meal together before trying to get a good night's sleep. On the Sunday we are up early and after tucking into a large breakfast we will head out to begin the hike up and down the mountain. A typical group will normally take about 7 hours in total to hike up and down the mountain with plenty of rest stops. Between April and October the café at the top is open where people can enjoy refreshments, use the toilets and possibly buy souvenirs in the gift shop. We will then travel back in the evening.

Scafell Pike

Scafell Pike is England's highest mountain at 978m (3,209ft) and is situated to the west of the Lake District National Park in North West England. We usually do the hike starting from Wasdale Head and it is a trip we can usually do any time of year. On the Saturday we would travel up and usually do a walk in the afternoon around the Coniston Water area where there are a selection of beautiful walks to choose from before going to the hotel, normally on the coast at Whitehaven. On the Sunday, after breakfast, we travel the short journey to the starting point of the hike at Wasdale Head and begin the walk. Typically it takes about 6 hours to reach the summit and back down, with plenty of rest breaks.

Helvellyn

The Helvellyn trip is similar to the Scafell Pike trip being in the Lake District National Park. It is perhaps the most popular mountain in the park and stands at 950m (3,117ft) tall, which makes it the third highest peak in England. On the Saturday afternoon we would usually do a picturesque walk in the Ullswater lake area before going to the hotel in the evening. On Sunday we do the hike up Helvellyn, typically starting from Patterdale, and if the weather is good we will go along the famous Striding Edge before looping round and coming down from the summit via Swirral Edge and returning to Glenridding. It is a fantastic walk and will usually take about 6 hours in total including plenty of breaks.

Ben Nevis

The 'Big Ben' is the highest mountain in the United Kingdom, standing at 1,344m (4,409ft) tall. It can be found in the North East of Scotland near to the town of Fort William. This trip requires two nights in a hotel due to the distance we have to travel. We usually stop on the way at the beautiful and stunning Loch Lomand for a short walk and break. Staying in Fort William it only takes about ten minutes to arrive at the starting point for the hike up to the summit. It is a long walk but if you are lucky with the weather then the views are spectacular. We usually allow 7–8 hours in total for the hike to the summit and back down, including plenty of stops. The effort is well worth it to stand on top of the nation's highest mountain, and then a celebratory meal can be enjoyed in the evening before travelling back the next day.

Brecon Beacons

Situated in mid-South Wales, the Brecon Beacons are a beautiful array of hills and mountains including some wonderful forests, rivers and waterfalls. On the Saturday we would do a walk of about 3 hours in total that will take in several stunning waterfalls, including one that you can actually walk behind, which is a strange but great feeling. Staying overnight at a nearby hotel the group will enjoy an evening meal and then on the Sunday we will do a longer walk of about 5 hours, including going up the highest peak in the Brecon Beacons, called Pen Y Fan, which stands at 886m (2,907ft) tall.

North Devon Coast

There are no mountains involved with this trip but there are some stunning coastal views and beautiful scenic paths. We travel down to North Devon on the Saturday and in the afternoon there are a few lovely short coastal walks to choose from, and some time to visit one or two of the coastal towns and harbours and enjoy a Devon Cream Tea!

On the Sunday the main walk goes from Ilfracombe to Woolacombe which is approximately 9 miles of wonderful coastal paths and cliffs with the occasional steep up and down section and a few chances to go on to the beaches. Passing through several small coastal villages and hamlets it is a beautiful walk lasting about 6 hours in total with stops and a picnic lunch. A little bit of time can be spent in Woolacombe, where there are huge sandy beaches, before the return travel back in the evening.

Yorkshire 3 Peaks Challenge

This is a tough but very satisfying challenge where you walk nearly 25 miles, including the three highest mountains in the North Yorkshire Dales. The aim is to complete the circular challenge in under 12 hours from start to finish, which is situated in the small village of Horton-in-Ribblesdale by the old post office and café.

A normal start time is before 7am in the morning if possible and the first mountain is Pen-y-Ghent, which you arrive at quite quickly; although the smallest of the three mountains it is the second steepest. Once the first mountain is completed there is a very long section towards Whernside, the tallest mountain and the second to be completed. Just before you start the ascent of Whernside there is the famous Ribblehead viaduct and also a welcome café van where the tea and bacon baps are recommended!

Whernside takes a long time to hike up but once achieved you just have the final mountain to go, called Ingleborough. There is another long walk until you reach the bottom of a very steep section and then at the top is a wide open area where the highest point and marker is in the far corner. Now all three mountains have been climbed and it's the long descent back to Horton-in-Ribblesdale, and you have completed a fantastic challenge. Throughout there are wonderful views and beautiful scenery and all the effort is worth it.

National 3 Peaks (sub 24hrs) Challenge

The National 3 Peaks Challenge takes in the highest mountains in England, Scotland and Wales, being Scafell Pike at 978m, Ben Nevis at 1,344m and Snowdon at 1,085m. We normally start with Snowdon and finish with Ben Nevis, which we have found is the best way for a number of different reasons.

We are able to enjoy a long lie-in on the Saturday before travelling up to Snowdon in the afternoon to start the actual challenge at about 6.30pm in the evening. From the Pen-y-Pass car park we take the Pyg track up and the Miners track down in 4 hours or less, so only the last part is in the dark. The drive to Scafell Pike takes about 4½ hours and we then commence the climb from Wasdale Head in the dark, but before we reach the summit the sun has risen and it is daylight. The climb up and down takes about 4 hours and then it is the long drive to Scotland for the final mountain. The drive usually takes about 5½ hours, so if everything has gone to plan it allows up to 6 hours to climb up and down Ben Nevis during the afternoon. Challenge complete and achieved and we can celebrate with a big meal and a few drinks before catching up on our sleep! After staying overnight in Fort William we than travel back the next day.

It is a great challenge and there is a wonderful sense of achievement in completing it, and despite what many people think you do not have to run or walk fast. The key is to maintain a steady, moderate pace and limit the number of stops and breaks to the minimum whilst walking. During the travel between mountains is the time to eat, drink, change clothes, relax, sleep, etc., so whilst climbing only small snacks and limited drinks are needed.

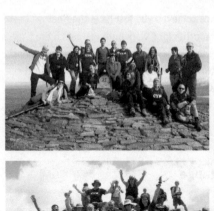

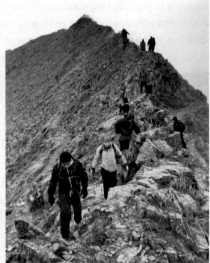

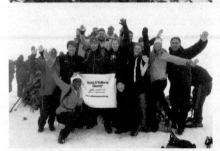

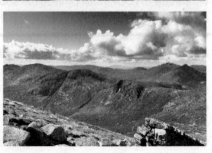

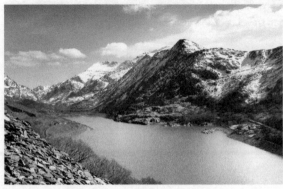

A selection of our UK trips including Helvellyn, Scafell Pike, Slieve Donard, Snowdon, Pen Y Fan, Helvellyn and Ben Nevis.

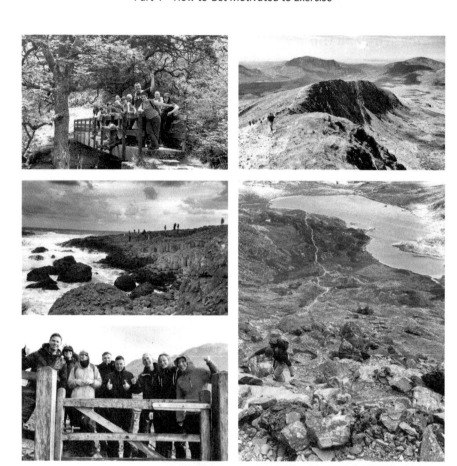

A selection of our UK trips including Snowdon, Brecon Beacons, Peak District, Ben Nevis and Giant's Causeway.

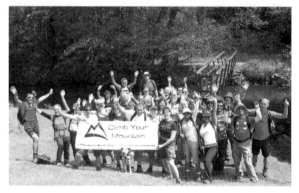

Northern Ireland trip

The highest peak in Northern Ireland is a mountain called Slieve Donard, which is situated close to the town of Newcastle, on the coast, a couple of hours south of Belfast. It is not that high at 850m (2,790ft); however, it does represent a good challenge and is comparable to other UK mountains like Snowdon and Scafell Pike. The whole area is lovely and the hike up to the summit provides some beautiful views and scenery; a realistic time up and down is about 6 hours in total.

Belfast is a great place to visit and very welcoming, with opportunities to enjoy some Irish music at the many pubs or visit the historic Titanic Experience down by the docks. There is also the option of travelling north of Belfast to the world famous Giant's Causeway, which is a unique and fascinating natural phenomenon on the coast overlooking the Irish Sea.

Overseas trips

There are several bigger overseas trips and challenges that we have taken, which are not only fantastic experiences for those taking part, they also provide essential funds for the charity. We hope that more people will be inspired and motivated to participate in these trips with and for our charity. Below is featured a selection of the trips available with an overview of each, and of course, please get in touch if you are interested in any of these.

Kilimanjaro

Mount Kilimanjaro is officially the world's highest free-standing mountain (i.e. not part of a mountain range). It is a dormant volcano situated in Tanzania, close to the Kenya border. Kilimanjaro itself consists of three volcanos – Mwenzi, Shira and Kibo, with Uhuru Peak being the highest part of Kibo and officially the highest point at 5,895m (19,330ft). There is no technical or difficult climbing involved, just walking, so anyone can potentially do this trip.

A typical trip will last for 10 days in total with 7 of the days on the mountain. A safari day, a trip to a local school, orphanage or Masai village are also included as part of the overall experience. There are a number of routes up and down Kilimanjaro though we usually use either Machame route or Rongai route to go up, and typically stay in Moshi, or sometimes Arusha.

Due to the height of Kilimanjaro and the altitude factor it is important to allow a steady ascent over 5 days minimum to allow your body to adjust and acclimatise effectively. Normally we would arrive at the summit base camp after five full days of trekking before embarking on the summit climb during the night. Most people will start the steep summit climb by midnight with the aim to reach the summit at Uhuru Peak close to sunrise or soon after a 6–8-hour slow and steady walk.

At the top of the mountain you can clearly see both the large crater of the volcano and also the huge ice glaciers that sit on top. From a distance as you start your Kilimanjaro journey the white stuff on top of the mountain looks like a bit of snow; however, as you stand next to these enormous white glaciers you cannot fail but feel in awe. At the summit is an official sign where you can take your photos and reflect on an exceptional achievement and experience.

Within a day and a half of trekking down the mountain you are back in Moshi celebrating with a cold beer or sugary fizzy drink, having a proper shower and enjoying the abundance of oxygen in the air. Africa is a wonderful experience and the effort of climbing Kilimanjaro is definitely worth it and the challenge is truly an achievement of a lifetime.

The Inca Trail and Machu Picchu

The ancient Inca settlement of Machu Picchu is considered one of the new Seven Wonders of the World and it really is an incredible site for a number of reasons. However, seeing Machu Picchu is simply the cherry on top of the icing on the cake if you also experience the full classic Inca Trail located in Peru on the South American continent.

First you fly in to Lima on the Pacific coast, the capital city of Peru, before next flying to the very picturesque town of Cusco that lies at over 3,000m above sea level. Due to the altitude you are likely to notice the thinning air and a couple of day's acclimatisation here is recommended. There are various historic and cultural places to visit nearby including the Saksaywaman site. You will also see many llamas and alpacas wherever you go.

The classic Inca Trail is a four-day trek through wonderful forests, jungles, mountain passes, old Inca ruins, farmlands and much more. The highest point you reach is called 'Dead Woman's Pass' at just over 4,200m before you drop down towards Machu Picchu, which lies at about 2,500m. You reach Machu Picchu from above, entering through the Sun Gate, and the sight you see on arrival is breathtaking.

Machu Picchu lies literally in the middle of nowhere, hidden by large mountains and forests all around. It is a vast, ancient village of the Incas and when the local Incas were conquered in the seventeenth century the site remained unseen by westerners until it was discovered in 1911 by an American explorer.

The trek itself is quite steep in places and you average about six hours' walking a day but the effort and scenery all around is definitely worth it. Peru and the Inca Trail offer a unique cultural experience, the people are remarkably humble, colourful and friendly and the landscape offers everything you would want to see.

Everest Base Camp and Kala Pattar

The Himalayas mountain range is an extraordinary and stunning natural phenomenon and only seeing it with your own eyes can you really capture the sheer size, scale and beauty of these magnificent mountains. The trip we do is the classical Everest Base Camp trek with the optional Kala Pattar mountain in order to get even better and closer views of Mount Everest.

From Kathmandu we take the short forty-five minute flight to Lukla Airport situated to the south of Everest and from there the official trek begins. Lukla lies at approximately 2,800m above sea level and over the next seven days we reach Base Camp at approximately 5,300m, and Kala Pattar is at 5,545m.

The trek is a wonderful mix of lush greenery, gigantic snow-capped mountains, small colourful villages and tea rooms, the incredible Dudh Kosi river, high rope bridges, monasteries, temples, prayer wheels, prayer flags, many yaks and many local Nepalese people carrying extraordinary amounts of goods on their back. The scenery is always breathtaking, as are some of the steep steps both up and down on the route as you meander your way slowly upwards and northwards towards Everest.

Although the altitude can be problematic, the relatively slow ascent means that issues are rare and most people only suffer very mild effects of the thinning air as they trek higher. The accommodation is a very good mix of permanent campsites and lodges in the small villages you go through in the region. The final settlement before base camp is Gorak Shep at 5,200m and it is a great opportunity to reflect on all the people who have been there before and the history of the place and region.

It takes about three hours from Gorak Shep to base camp which is simply an area alongside the Khumba glacier and at the base of the icefall. There is an official place representing base camp for photographs and celebrations, though. From Kala Pattar you are rewarded with amazing views of Everest which you don't actually get from base camp so it is worth the extra effort.

Kathmandu is definitely an experience worth seeing and exploring. Many temples, world heritage sites, cultural experiences and markets sit within the poverty-stricken areas and overcrowded, dusty streets and roads, but the city is always vibrant and colourful.

The Great Wall of China

The Great Wall of China covers a few thousand miles in total across the country, but you will spend five or six days walking several sections, including both more modern restored parts and old unrestored sections of the wall. Arriving in Beijing, the modern motorways mean that the journey to the start of the trek is only about two hours, but you will feel as if you are in a different country, because the contrast between Beijing and the small country villages is enormous.

Each day on the trek you will walk along different sections, which will vary in height and steepness as you go from one tower to another with fantastic views all around. An average day may include up to six hours of walking, some of it quite challenging, though you will have plenty of time to rest, stop and visit some of the small villages, tea rooms and shops. Overnight you will stay in either excellent campsites or small lodges, both of which are comfortable and in very scenic locations.

After the trek you will be able to enjoy the very contrasting experience of Beijing, which has a unique mix of modern and historic buildings and atmosphere. It is a great city

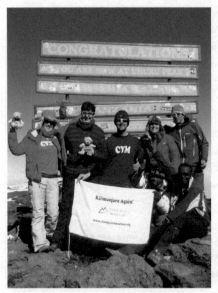
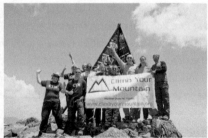
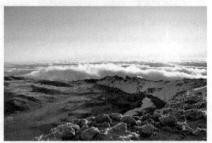
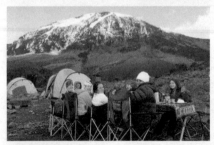
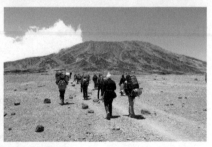
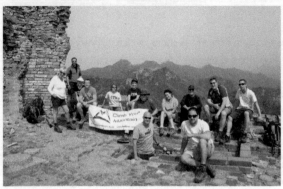

A selection of our overseas challenges including Kilimanjaro, Mount Toubkal and the Great Wall of China.

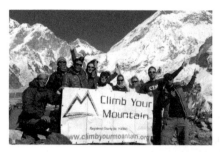

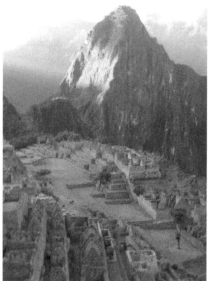

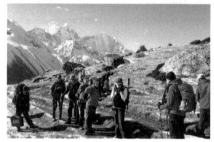

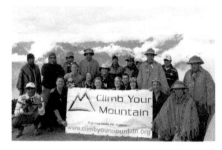

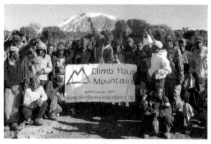

A selection of our overseas challenges including Kilimanjaro, Everest Base Camp and the Inca Trail.

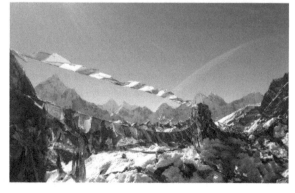

to experience with lots to see and places to go to including Tiananmen Square, the Forbidden City and the Olympic Stadium. The trip is a wonderful cultural and historic experience and you get a real insight into the modern and the old China.

Mount Toubkal

Situated in Morocco, Mount Toubkal is the highest mountain in the Atlas range of mountains, reaching a height of 4,167m above sea level. Although there are several longer options and routes it is possible to hike up and down the mountain in just three days and two nights.

You fly to Marrakesh, the large vibrant city in the heart of Morocco and from there travel to Imil to begin the ascent of the mountain. The hiking can be quite strenuous at times and the altitude will be noticeable to most people but the scenery makes up for this and it feels like a proper mountain. You will find a few small shops and tea rooms along the route and there is a wonderful large, old refuge building close to where you begin the second day summit climb.

At the summit you will be able to see for miles, with other peaks visible across the extensive Atlas mountain range. You will see a few other hikers and lots of mountain goats but otherwise it is a very quiet, peaceful location and feels quite remote, in a good way. Once back down you can then enjoy the hustle and bustle of Marrakesh, including the large market square and surrounding streets and buildings.

Running Challenges

There are so many potential running challenges you could do, from a 5k race through to marathons and even ultra-marathons. No matter how much of a runner you currently are, nearly everyone has the potential to train and improve and successfully complete a running challenge. The training will be very beneficial in a number of ways and the event itself will be like a huge cherry on top of the cake! Completing a running challenge is so rewarding as you battle against yourself, give it your all and then collect your medal.

There are so many events to choose from, including local races through to major events all across the world. I have been fortunate to run marathons in New York, Las Vegas, Toronto and Rotterdam as well as many marathons in the UK and they are always fantastic experiences and very beneficial. Even better would be to do a running challenge for CYM and raise money for our charity!

Walking Challenges

Perhaps running isn't for you or you would prefer to do a walking challenge, and the good news is that there are more and more big, well-organised walking challenges appearing all the time. For example, there is the Grand Union Canal Walk and the Great Thames Path Walk which are both 100 kilometres in distance (although you can choose to do less!). Challenging yourself to walk for such long distances is tough but also very rewarding and as with any challenge the effort is rewarded by the sense of achievement and pride you can feel.

The more training you can do the better and ensuring you have good footwear and socks is essential. Even if you are very active and consider yourself very fit, a long-distance walking challenge will test you and is definitely a great different option for you to try. Plus if you don't consider yourself fit then walking helps to level the playing field and you can participate in a great challenge without being intimidated by the 'super fit' people! And again, even better if you take part in one of these long-distance walking challenges and raise money for our charity.

If you are interested in any of these challenges or have some ideas of your own then please get in touch as I would love to hear from you. Any money raised or donated would be very much appreciated and would enable us to produce more books, videos, courses and workshops for more people. Please email info@climbyourmountain.org

Summary and Moving Forward

We are born to be active

It is important to remember and appreciate that as humans we are born to be active. Think about how natural young children seem when playing and running about and how our bodies are designed with physical activity being a key factor for our evolution as a species. Also think about the fact if we stop doing what we have evolved to do and what our body is meant to do then it makes sense that there are consequences to our health.

Why we don't exercise

There are many reasons and excuses why we don't exercise or are as physically active as we should be. Overall it comes down to choices; exercise is often seen as the harder choice so many people do not opt for it. Many people do not understand the consequences of not being physically active and see exercise as a luxury or something they may fit in every now and then if they have some spare time. By treating it as such a low priority, then if other things come up, or if they are feeling tired or it isn't convenient then more often than not people don't exercise.

Physiological and mental health benefits of exercise

Being more physically active will almost certainly help to improve your confidence and self-esteem, reduce stress and anxiety as well as helping to prevent, manage or treat depression. The positive effect on the brain through regulating and boosting neurotransmitters also comes with no side effects or stigmas attached. Other areas like alertness, learning and memory will benefit and attention deficit hyperactivity disorder and addictive behaviour can be greatly improved through exercise.

Behavioural benefits of exercise

You are likely to find that by being more physically active you will have more energy and be more productive. You are also likely to sleep better, which in turn helps you to feel more energised, positive and happier. You will probably make new friends and go to new places by being more socially engaged and active and your self-worth and personal pride will increase by doing exercise and activities that you know are good for you, are fulfilling and can offer a sense of achievement.

Physical benefits of exercise

There is such a wide range of physical health benefits that can result from doing exercise. Externally you can lose weight, tone up, develop more muscle and reduce fat, plus your skin and hair condition can improve. Internally your blood pressure and bad cholesterol levels can be lowered, your arteries opened, your lung capacity increased and your chances of heart disease and related issues decreased. Also your risk of developing several cancers and other serious illness can be significantly reduced by being more physically active.

How to get motivated to exercise

It can be very difficult to get motivated to exercise, especially if you are not used to being physically active and haven't experienced the range of benefits exercise can bring. It's important to try to understand what motivates and demotivates you and why, and then how you can become more motivated. The more you understand the easier it will become and the likelihood then is that the more you do exercise the more motivated you will become anyway, so it forms a very positive virtuous circle in that respect.

Challenge yourself

A great way to boost your confidence, feel happier, do more exercise and be more motivated is to set yourself a challenge or some challenges. By pushing yourself in this way you will benefit from seeing what you are capable of, experiencing the challenge, being fulfilled, feeling proud and enjoying the sense of achievement it brings. Think about what challenges you could participate in, what goals you could set yourself and perhaps think about joining in with some of the CYM Challenges too!

I hope you have found the book informative, interesting and beneficial. I also hope it has motivated you to become more active, do more exercise and lead a healthier and happier life. Feel free to get in contact and perhaps I will see you on some future CYM trips and challenges!

'The way to get started is to quit talking and begin doing.' – *Walt Disney*

About the
'Climb Your Mountain' Charity

The Climb Your Mountain (CYM) charity was set up in 2008 by Charlie Wardle with the aim of helping anyone who felt they had their own personal mountain to climb in life. CYM offers advice, support, information, education, activities and opportunities for people to help themselves improve their health and happiness and effectively climb their own personal mountain.

Everyone will go through difficult times in life which may include work issues, relationship problems, financial pressures, health concerns, low confidence, anxiety, depression, social isolation, bereavement, etc., and Climb Your Mountain (CYM) offers a range of opportunities for people to help them through these difficult times in a number of ways.

CYM Health offers a range of free practical, easy-to-read, informative self-help books, as well as free online video workshops on the same topics for people to view and benefit from. Charlie Wardle also delivers talks, seminars, courses and workshops to the general public and to companies on a range of health and wellbeing topics.

To fund the charity and be able to offer all the free CYM Health services, the CYM Challenges division offers a range of fantastic trips and challenges across the UK and also some overseas trips. Anyone can participate in these great-value trips and challenges and have an amazing experience whilst also helping to support and fund the charity.

To find out more about the 'Climb Your Mountain' charity:

Website www.climbyourmountain.org

Email info@climbyourmountain.org

We rely heavily for funding on people making donations and raising money from taking part in trips and challenges. If you can help by making a donation please go to

www.justgiving.com/climbym

or get in touch and take part in a trip or challenge with us!

You can also TEXT a £5 donation to the charity

TEXT: BOOK32£5

To: 70070

Or an online donation via:

www.justgiving.com/healthbooks

THANK YOU!